Learning Activities in Psychiatric Nursing

Learning Activities in Psychiatric Nursing

Holly Skodol Wilson, R.N., Ph.D.

Carol Ren Kneisl, R.N., M.S.

ADDISON-WESLEY PUBLISHING COMPANY
Medical/Nursing Division, Menlo Park, California
Reading, Massachusetts · London · Amsterdam
Don Mills, Ontario · Sydney

ISBN 0-201-08342-6
EFGHIJKLMN-AL-89876543210

Library of Congress Catalog Card Number 78-7775

ADDISON-WESLEY PUBLISHING COMPANY
Medical/Nursing Division
2725 Sand Hill Road
Menlo Park, California 94025

Preface

Teachers of psychiatric nursing have repeatedly expressed the need for a resource that combines in one volume the many and varied guides and structured learning activities energetically sought, painstakingly developed anew, and customarily used in one form or another to teach psychiatric nursing content. We have written this workbook to fill the gap and to bring important concepts, theories, and skills alive for students and faculty alike.

The workbook has been designed as a satellite to our text *Psychiatric Nursing.* It shares the premises of that text—that psychiatric nurses have as their central concern the humanity of people, that people search for meaning in their interactions with others, and that people change themselves, their worlds, and their destinies as they engage in social dialogue. The text and this workbook are specifically intended to reflect a holistic nursing philosophy and to suit nursing curricula based on *nursing* concepts rather than borrowed medical models.

UNIQUE FEATURES

The workbook consists of a compendium of action-oriented heuristics or learning activities in which students practice using ideas and strategies covered in depth in the text. Through individual and small group exercises, inventories, simulations, assessment tools, and questionnaires, the theory-practice connection is promoted. Students actually live through, or experience, the interpersonal phenomena they have read or heard about. Learning is enhanced through this experiential mode.

Although designed for students of psychiatric nursing, the book's contents are appropriate to nursing in every setting, whenever and wherever interpersonal and human relations concepts are applied. In addition to learning theory and practice specific to psychiatric nursing, students will learn about values, how they influence nursing care, and how personal attributes influence the role of each nurse.

Large portions of this book can be used in courses on small group dynamics, group psychotherapy, and other specific topics. Some tools have multiple purposes—that is, the same tool can be used, for example, to focus on the role of values in nursing behavior and on the process of decision making by consensus, at the option of the individual teacher.

While the workbook has been prepared as a companion to the text and is keyed to text chapters at appropriate places, it can readily be used alone or with an alternative text with minimal sequencing.

LEVEL OF THE BOOK

Workbooks are generally directed to the needs of a single level of students. This one, on the contrary, is geared to all levels of students and to practitioners of nursing as well. The tools and activities are appropriate to both undergraduate and graduate nursing curricula, depending on the depth and breadth of responses expected of the students. They may also be used selectively in in-service education programs for nursing practitioners.

USING THE BOOK TO FULL ADVANTAGE

This workbook is one element of a three-part set. The three components—workbook, instructor's guide, and text—form a complete package for teaching psychiatric nursing theoretical and clinical content, either as a separate course or as an integrated thread in a nursing curriculum.

The text is a contemporary and comprehensive approach to the content and concepts of psychiatric nursing, emphasizing a holistic approach. The instructor's guide, keyed to the text chapter by chapter, offers the teacher all the customary materials required in nursing course syllabi, including measurable behavioral objectives, topical lecture outlines, higher order questions for seminar and conference discussion, references to the complementary learning activities in the workbook, and test items.

Each exercise, inventory, simulation, assessment tool, and questionnaire in the workbook is thoroughly explained, to minimize the coordination tasks of the instructor. An instructor with a large group of students can thus have them work in several small groups independently, for enhanced learning and discussion. Students and faculty can easily locate all the materials that each structured learning activity requires. Theoretical background for each tool is available in the text.

Tear-away sheets are provided so that students can complete experiences on their own and turn the sheets in to the instructor for review. It is recommended that instructors review each learning activity before assigning it, to determine how to use it most effectively. Some are designed as intrapersonal exercises, which the individual student may choose to share with the instructor or with peers. It is suggested that the choice to share be left to the student, to allow for personal privacy and to encourage greater honesty in answering questions. Other tools may be used in dyads, triads, or small groups. The instructor may wish to bring all students together for a discussion period, as well. Guidelines for discussion have been provided for appropriate tools.

Some of the exercises and inventories may produce anxiety or be stressful for students. In those cases, supportive action by the instructor may be helpful.

ORGANIZATION OF MATERIALS

Students and faculty will find a wide array of useful classroom and clinical tools here. Part I focuses on the psychiatric nurse as a person. Our intent is to help students identify how they deal with and influence the social dialogues they have with others. The learning activities in this part are concerned with person-as-nurse relationships and experiences in nursing practice.

The assessment exercises presented in part 2 concern the search for meaning in human interaction. They encourage the nurse to solve problems and make decisions based on systematically collected data rather than preconceived interpretations of the experiences of others.

Part 3 contains learning activities in which students practice psychiatric nursing interventions. These tools provide simulated situations, directions, and a structured format for feedback and interaction with peers and faculty.

ACKNOWLEDGMENTS

We thank Marilyn Sanderson, Betty Inzinna, and Debbie Bucki, psychiatric nursing clinical specialists, who provided verbatim data from individual, group, marital couple, and family therapy sessions for the analysis exercises.

Carol Szalasny and Sally Cochran took on the unenviable task of typing the manuscript from our handwritten and cut-and-paste drafts and did their usual superb job.

Undergraduates and faculty members at Sonoma State College and graduate students in the Community Psychiatric Nursing Program at State University of New York at Buffalo tested our tools, and their critiques account for significant refinements in the book.

Contents

PART I

The Person as Psychiatric Nurse

Beliefs about "Mental Illness"

DIRECTIONS

The following statements reflect ideas and beliefs about conditions that are labeled "mental illness" and about people who become "mental patients." Rate each with a score ranging from 5 to 0, based on the following scale:

5 Strongly agree   2 Not sure but probably disagree

4 Agree   1 Disagree

3 Not sure but probably agree   0 Strongly disagree

There are no right or wrong answers, so be as honest as you can.

___4___ 1. When you have a problem or worry, it is better not to think about it but rather keep busy with more pleasant things.

___1___ 2. All clients in mental hospitals should be prevented by a painless operation from having children.

___1___ 3. One of the main causes of mental illness is a lack of moral strength or will power.

___3___ 4. Every person should have complete faith in some supernatural power whose decisions he or she obeys without question.

___3___ 5. Although some mental clients seem all right, it is dangerous to forget for a moment that they are mentally ill.

___3___ 6. Even though clients in mental hospitals behave in funny ways, it is wrong to laugh about them.

___2___ 7. Clients in mental hospitals are in many ways like children.

Source: Adapted from items in Jacob Cohen and E. L. Struening, "Opinions about Mental Illness Scale," *Journal of Abnormal and Social Psychology* 64 (1962): 349-60. Copyright 1962 by the American Psychological Association. Reprinted by permission.

___2___ 8. Our mental hospitals seem more like prisons than like places where mentally ill people can be cared for.

___2___ 9. Although they usually aren't aware of it, many people become mentally ill to avoid the difficult problems of everyday life.

___3___ 10. More tax money should be spent in the care and treatment of people with severe mental illness.

___4___ 11. Many mental clients are capable of skilled labor, even though in some ways they are very disturbed mentally.

___3___ 12. Many people who have never been clients in a mental hospital are more mentally ill than many hospitalized mental clients.

___2___ 13. Many mental clients would remain in the hospital until they were well even if the doors were unlocked.

___3___ 14. The clients of a mental hospital should have something to say about the way the hospital is run.

___3___ 15. More tax money should be spent in the care and treatment of people with severe mental illness.

___1___ 16. A woman would be foolish to marry a man who has had a severe mental illness, even though he seems fully recovered.

___2___ 17. People who have been clients in a mental hospital will never be their old selves again.

___2___ 18. Small children should not be allowed to visit their parents who are clients in mental hospitals.

___2___ 19. Most clients in mental hospitals don't care how they look.

___2___ 20. Anyone who is in a hospital for a mental illness should not be allowed to vote.

___3___ 21. Mental clients come from homes where the parents took little interest in their children.

___2___ 22. The mental illness of many people is caused by the separation or divorce of their parents during childhood.

___3___ 23. If parents loved their children more, there would be less mental illness.

___3___ 24. If the children of normal parents were raised by mentally ill parents, they would probably become mentally ill.

___2___ 25. People who are successful in their work seldom become mentally ill.

EXPLANATION OF SCORING

Five attitude orientations are represented in the above twenty-five items. Each scale is scored separately. Add your individual scores for attitude items 1-5, 6-10, 11-15, 16-20, and 21-25. Total scores for each scale can range from a high of 25 to a low of 0.

Scale A   *Authoritarianism* (items 1-5). These items reflect a view of the mentally ill as an inferior class requiring coercive handling.

Scale B   *Benevolence* (6-10). This scale reflects a kindly paternalistic view of patients, with emphasis on religion and humanism rather than science.

Scale C   *Mental Hygiene Ideology* (11-15). This reflects an orientation that embodies the tenets of modern mental health professionals and the mental hygiene movement.

Scale D   *Social Restrictiveness* (16-20). The key belief here is that mentally ill people are a threat to society, particularly the family, and therefore must be restricted in their functioning.

Scale E   *Interpersonal Etiology* (21-25). This scale reflects the belief that mental illness arises from interpersonal experience, especially deprivation of parental love during childhood.

To profile your results, draw a line through each row of the chart below at the point on the row that represents your score. Shade in in the area between zero and the line you have drawn in each row.

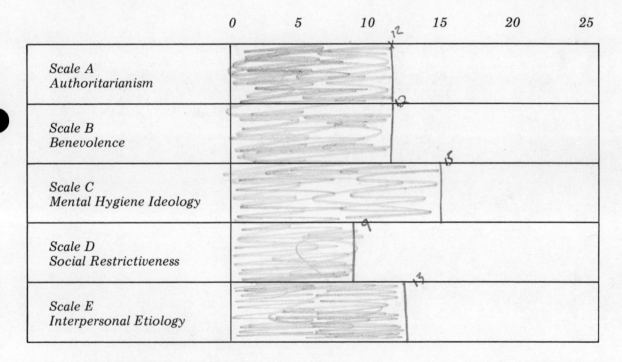

DISCUSSION GUIDE

After each of you has arrived at a total score for each scale, discuss the five scales by name, considering these questions:

1. What in your own life experience might have led to the dominance of one attitude orientation or another?

2. Would you have predicted the scales on which you received high scores?

3. How might your attitudes influence your interactions and effectiveness with psychiatric clients?

4. How do terms such as *willpower*, *mentally ill*, etc., affect your judgment?

Psychiatric Nursing Ideology Scale

DIRECTIONS

The following statements reflect ideas and beliefs about psychiatric nursing and what psychiatric nurses should do in their practice. Rate each with a score ranging from 5 to 0, based on the following scale:

5 Strongly agree

4 Agree

3 Not sure but probably agree

2 Not sure but probably disagree

1 Disagree

0 Strongly disagree

___2___ 1. Drugs are the most effective form of treatment for emotionally disturbed persons.

___3___ 2. The psychiatric nurse should function as an agent for social change.

___1___ 3. Psychiatric nurses can be more effective working indirectly with large numbers of clients than working intensively with small numbers of clients.

___1___ 4. In inpatient settings, somatic forms of treatment tend to be more effective than milieu therapy or psychotherapy.

___4___ 5. Working relations among members of the mental health professions would probably improve considerably if all professionals addressed each other by first name.

___4___ 6. Psychotherapy reflects greater respect for the client as an individual than any other form of treatment.

___2___ 7. Most hospitalized clients should be strongly encouraged to become actively involved in the treatment of other clients on their unit.

___4___ 8. The psychiatric nurse is responsible for the emotionally disturbed person who does not seek the nurse out, as well as for the one who does.

___3___ 9. The treatment of the mentally ill cannot be expected to improve materially until the neurological and biochemical bases for mental illness are better understood.

___2___ 10. One of the main problems in mental health care is that intensive one-to-one psychotherapy is not used enough.

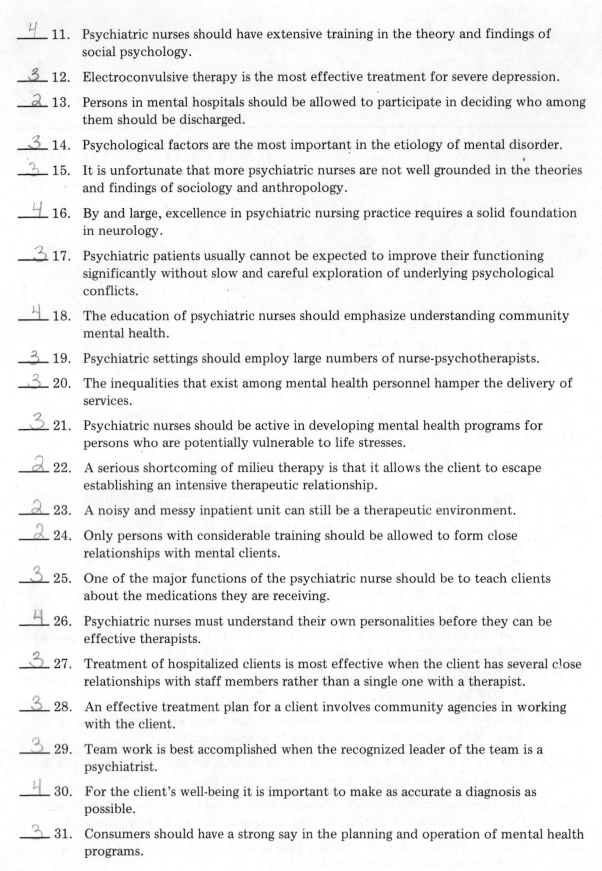

___4___ 11. Psychiatric nurses should have extensive training in the theory and findings of social psychology.

___3___ 12. Electroconvulsive therapy is the most effective treatment for severe depression.

___2___ 13. Persons in mental hospitals should be allowed to participate in deciding who among them should be discharged.

___3___ 14. Psychological factors are the most important in the etiology of mental disorder.

___3___ 15. It is unfortunate that more psychiatric nurses are not well grounded in the theories and findings of sociology and anthropology.

___4___ 16. By and large, excellence in psychiatric nursing practice requires a solid foundation in neurology.

___3___ 17. Psychiatric patients usually cannot be expected to improve their functioning significantly without slow and careful exploration of underlying psychological conflicts.

___4___ 18. The education of psychiatric nurses should emphasize understanding community mental health.

___3___ 19. Psychiatric settings should employ large numbers of nurse-psychotherapists.

___3___ 20. The inequalities that exist among mental health personnel hamper the delivery of services.

___3___ 21. Psychiatric nurses should be active in developing mental health programs for persons who are potentially vulnerable to life stresses.

___2___ 22. A serious shortcoming of milieu therapy is that it allows the client to escape establishing an intensive therapeutic relationship.

___2___ 23. A noisy and messy inpatient unit can still be a therapeutic environment.

___2___ 24. Only persons with considerable training should be allowed to form close relationships with mental clients.

___3___ 25. One of the major functions of the psychiatric nurse should be to teach clients about the medications they are receiving.

___4___ 26. Psychiatric nurses must understand their own personalities before they can be effective therapists.

___3___ 27. Treatment of hospitalized clients is most effective when the client has several close relationships with staff members rather than a single one with a therapist.

___3___ 28. An effective treatment plan for a client involves community agencies in working with the client.

___3___ 29. Team work is best accomplished when the recognized leader of the team is a psychiatrist.

___4___ 30. For the client's well-being it is important to make as accurate a diagnosis as possible.

___3___ 31. Consumers should have a strong say in the planning and operation of mental health programs.

___4___ 32. An inpatient psychiatric facility is only one part of a comprehensive mental health program for a community.

EXPLANATION OF SCORING

Four ideological orientations are represented in the above thirty-two items. Each scale is scored separately. Add your individual scores for the items listed under each scale below. Total scores for each scale can range from a high of 40 to a low of 0.

Scale A *Medical Model Ideology* (items 1, 4, 9, 12, 16, 25, 29, 30). These items reflect a view based on an illness model that emphasizes somatic therapy. (23)

Scale B *Milieu Therapy Ideology* (items 5, 7, 11, 13, 15, 20, 23, 27). This scale represents the belief that the psychiatric hospital as a social system, rather than the individual, is the subject of analysis and intervention. (23)

Scale C *Psychotherapist/Counselor Ideology* (items 6, 10, 14, 17, 19, 22, 24, 26). This scale focuses on psychotherapy as a specific treatment for specific psychological trauma and emphasizes the individual therapist-client relationship. (23)

Scale D *Community Mental Health Ideology* (items 2, 3, 8, 18, 21, 28, 31, 32). These items reflect an orientation toward social action as a means of promoting mental health and the treatment of mental illness in total populations. (25)

To profile your results, draw a line through each row of the chart below at the point on the row that represents your score. Shade in the area between zero and the line you have drawn in each row.

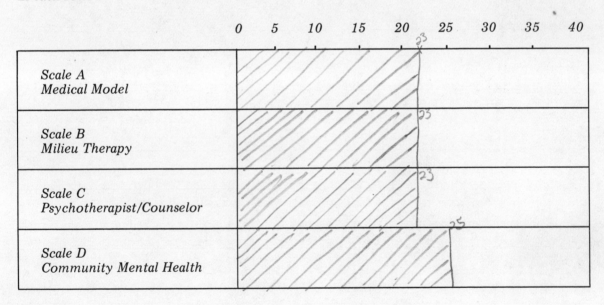

DISCUSSION GUIDE

After each of you has arrived at a total score for the four ideological orientations, discuss them by name, considering such questions as:

1. What in your life and professional experience might have led to the dominance of one psychiatric nursing ideology over another?

2. Would you have predicted the scales on which you received high scores?

3. How might your ideological orientations influence your interactions and effectiveness with psychiatric clients?

4. Which orientations do you feel are humanistic in nature?

Escape from Primavera Island

Primavera, a small island in the Pacific Ocean "ring of fire" (the circular area on the globe that contains most of the world's volcanoes and active earthquake activity), has been devastated by the unexpected eruption of an undersea volcano, which arose just off its west shore. Twelve survivors on the island have just received warning, by shortwave radio, of a *tsunami*, an oceanic tidal wave created by the unusual earthquakes and volcanic activity in this area of the Pacific. The tsunami is expected to reach Primavera in one hour. Its force and height will completely engulf and submerge the small, flat island. One helicopter has been dispatched to Primavera to rescue the survivors. Because of the distance between Primavera and other land masses, this is the only helicopter that will be able to reach it before the tsunami hits. There are no ships in the immediate area. The Sikorsky F77 helicopter can carry six passengers. Overloaded, it will probably be able to carry an absolute maximum of eight. Thus there will be room for seven passengers at the most, plus the pilot.

DIRECTIONS

Your group has only one hour to decide which seven of the twelve survivors on Primavera will escape the certain death the tsunami will bring. You must reach a decision before the tsunami reaches Primavera, or *all* will be lost. The twelve people are:

1. Samantha Spencer, nineteen, a former Miss Teenage America; enrolled in the drama department of a southern California university

2. Dr. Henry Spencer, forty-three, a marine biologist conducting a research study on Primavera; Nobel Prize recipient

3. Mrs. Renee Spencer, forty-one, housewife and mother

4. Bobby Spencer, thirteen, the youngest Spencer child; mentally retarded

5. Rhonda MacDougall, thirty-three, the owner and director of a multi-million-dollar company, which she built from a $4,000 investment seven years ago

6. Captain Vasily Piotrovich, fifty-nine, the captain of a Russian trawler thought to contain sophisticated spying equipment

7. Ludmila Zapotochny, forty-one, first mate and medical officer on the Russian trawler

8. Luis Jimenez, twenty-three, assistant chef at the only hotel on Primavera; the homosexual lover of Karl Sorensen

9. Karl Sorensen, thirty-four, Danish-born maitre d' at the hotel restaurant; Luis Jimenez's roommate and lover

10. Rabbi Sholom Klein, fifty, rabbi of the largest temple in the Northern Hemisphere

11. Arnella Jones, twenty-nine, Jamaican-born hotel maid; an ex-convict

12. Jean-Baptiste Jones, six-week-old son of Arnella Jones

DISCUSSION GUIDELINES

After each of you has identified your choices for the seven survivors, engage in a discussion that considers the following questions:

1. Whom did you select to survive?

2. What were your reasons for the choices?

3. How much agreement and disagreement did you find among your choices?

4. How do you feel about yourselves in relation to this exercise?

5. What values do the choices reflect?

4

Staff-Hiring Exercise

DIRECTIONS

You are the director of nursing service of a community hospital in a medium-sized western city. You must immediately replace a very fine intensive care unit staff nurse who died quite suddenly. You must make a choice from among four applicants—Donna, Harriet, Jim, and Beth. From personnel research and interviewing you have learned the following about them:

1. Donna had an exceptional academic record in a baccalaureate nursing program. She is bright and hard working, well liked and well mannered, but she is a very stubborn young woman. She is also a confirmed atheist and does not hide her lack of religious belief. When asked if she intended to meet the spiritual needs of patients and families, she replied that she would do what she believed and that no one had the right to ask her not to. The personnel administrator contends that the hospital owes a duty to the public not to approve a new nurse who holds fanatical ideas about atheism. Donna counters that an employer cannot discriminate against a person on the basis of religion or lack of religion in the United States. She maintains that, if she is qualified, she should be hired.

2. Harriet had an average academic record at a small diploma school of nursing. Her recommendations are just adequate, indicating clearly that some question about her competence remains in the minds of her teachers. When asked how well her previous practice had gone, Harriet replied that she did not finish administering all the care she was supposed to give. The personnel administrator contends that Harriet would be incompetent. Harriet asserts that she is willing and able to learn as she practices.

3. Jim had an exceptional academic record at a large, well-respected, private university. His recommendations were excellent as far as academic preparation was concerned. Jim is well liked by all and well mannered, but he definitely prefers the company of men to that of women. When questioned about this Jim acknowledged that it was true and that he was a homosexual, but he asserted that he had the situation in full control. Jim said that he would not allow any of his homosexual views to influence the performance of his

Source: Reprinted with permission of Macmillan Publishing Co., Inc. from COMMUNICATION GAMES by Karen R. Krupar. Copyright ©1973 by The Free Press, a Division of Macmillan Publishing Co., Inc.

role, but, if asked, would acknowledge them. The personnel administrator contends that the hospital has a responsibility to protect its patients from deviants and that exposure to Jim might be a detriment and an injury to patients. Jim contends that his sexual preference is his private life. He has his own circle of friends in a town fifty miles away. He has never been in trouble with the police during four years of undergraduate work and his previous work experiences. He maintains that he is well qualified and that his qualifications should be the basis for his employment.

4. Beth had a sporadic academic record from a large public university. The personnel administrator reports that she is neat, clean, and well dressed. She was a campus radical and took part in several protests, on one occasion spending eighteen days in jail because of her activities. Her record also shows that Beth has strong political leanings toward communism. Upon questioning, Beth admitted her association with certain violent political factions, but she assured the interviewer that she was now ready to settle down. She stressed that she would like to practice on the intensive care unit. The personnel administrator contends that the hospital cannot afford to subject its patients to a Communist. Beth maintains that her political views have nothing to do with her nursing qualifications and that she should be considered for the position.

Which candidate should you select to fill the position?

DISCUSSION GUIDELINES

After each of you has made a choice of a candidate, divide into groups of about five, and discuss the following questions:

1. Did you find the choice difficult? Why or why not?
2. Were any candidates easy to eliminate?
3. What process did you undergo in reaching a decision?
4. What did you learn about yourself and your values from your process and final decision?

Interpersonal Patterns Description

The following exercise focuses on your interactions with other individuals. It may help you think about how you behave when you initiate a relationship with another person or how you act in a group.

DIRECTIONS

The twenty verbs listed below describe some of the ways people feel and act from time to time. Think of your behavior in interactions with other people. How do you feel and act with them? Check the five verbs that you feel best describe your behavior in interactions with others.

_____ acquiesces	_____ disapproves
_____ advises	_____ evades
_____ agrees	_____ initiates
_____ analyzes	_____ judges
_____ assists	_____ leads
_____ concedes	_____ obliges
_____ cooperates	_____ relinquishes
_____ coordinates	_____ resists
_____ criticizes	_____ retreats
_____ directs	_____ withdraws

Source: David W. Johnson and Frank P. Johnson, JOINING TOGETHER: Group Theory and Group Skills, ©1975, pp. 46-47. Adapted by permission of Prentice-Hall, Inc., Englewood Cliffs, New Jersey.

EXPLANATION OF SCORING

There are two underlying factors or traits in the list of verbs: *dominance* (authority or control) and *sociability* (intimacy or friendliness). Most people tend either to like to control things (high dominance) or to let others control things (low dominance). Similarly most people tend either to be very warm and personal (high sociability) or to be somewhat cold and impersonal (low sociability). In the following boxes circle the five verbs you picked to describe yourself on the checklist. The box in which you circled three or more verbs represents your interpersonal pattern tendency.

	HIGH DOMINANCE	LOW DOMINANCE
HIGH SOCIABILITY	advises coordinates directs initiates leads	acquiesces agrees assists cooperates obliges
LOW SOCIABILITY	analyzes criticizes disapproves judges resists	concedes evades relinquishes retreats withdraws

DISCUSSION GUIDELINES

Divide into groups of three. Share with the other two members of your triad the results of the exercise, and ask whether they perceive you the way the results indicate. Discuss the following questions together:

1. What does your interpersonal pattern tendency say about you?

2. How might your interpersonal pattern tendency influence your interactions with clients, colleagues, professors, and supervisors?

3. If the other members of your triad perceive you differently from your perceptions of yourself, what might this indicate?

How Assertive Are You?

This assertiveness tool, although not a validated psychological scale or test, can help you assess your assertiveness. Be honest in your responses.

DIRECTIONS

Next to each statement below, write the number that describes you best, based on the following scale:

0 No or never

1 Somewhat or sometimes

2 About half the time

3 Usually or quite often

4 Almost always or entirely

__4__ 1. When a friend has borrowed my psychiatric nursing textbook and failed to return it as promised, I ask her or him about it.

__3__ 2. I am reluctant to insist that my household mate assumes her or his share of housekeeping tasks.

__2__ 3. When angry, I am likely to use obscenities.

__3__ 4. It disturbs me to have someone observe my clinical work with clients.

__0__ 5. When someone cuts in line ahead of me, I protest directly to the person.

__3__ 6. When another person's smoking disturbs me, I am reluctant to tell the person.

__4__ 7. I am comfortable giving compliments and praising others.

__4__ 8. I find myself saying "I'm sorry" when I don't really mean it.

__4__ 9. I am reluctant to describe myself positively to others.

__4__ 10. I feel uncomfortable making comments or asking questions in class.

__1__ 11. When I differ with a physician I respect, I speak up for my point of view.

___3___ 12. If a person criticizes me unfairly I am likely either to hit the person or to leave feeling angry and upset, rather than defend myself verbally.

___1___ 13. At a party I am likely to introduce myself and start a conversation with someone I don't know.

___1___ 14. I find myself shouting or crying when others don't go along with me.

___1___ 15. When my restaurant meal is not prepared or served as it should be, I ask the waiter or waitress to correct the situation.

___2___ 16. I find myself speaking for others or making decisions for them.

___2___ 17. When I am talking with someone I am able to maintain eye contact with that person.

___2___ 18. I am able to refuse a friend a favor if I don't wish to do what my friend asks of me.

___0___ 19. When a salesperson waits on someone before me who came to the counter after me, I can call attention to it.

___1___ 20. I "fly off the handle."

EXPLANATION OF SCORING

These questions assess assertive versus nonassertive or aggressive behavior. Assertive behavior is self-enhancing, goal-achieving behavior, freely chosen by the person, that honestly expresses that person's feelings. Nonassertive behavior denies the self, inhibits the expression of the person's feelings, allows others to choose for the self, and fails to achieve the individual's desired goals. Aggressive behavior accomplishes the person's own ends, is self-enhancing, and expresses feelings but at the expense of others, thus diminishing the other's freedom of choice and sense of worth.

For some questions in this tool, the assertive end of the scale is 0. For others it is 4. The key below tells you which behaviors are at the ends of the scales.

QUESTION	0 END OF SCALE	4 END OF SCALE
1-4	nonassertive	assertive ✓
2-3	assertive	nonassertive ✗
3-2	assertive ✓	aggressive
4-3	assertive	nonassertive ✗
5-0	nonassertive ✗	assertive
6-3	assertive	nonassertive ✗
7-4	nonassertive	assertive ✓
8-4	assertive	nonassertive ✗
9-4	assertive	nonassertive ✗
10-4	assertive	nonassertive ✗
11-1	nonassertive ✗	assertive
12-3	assertive	aggressive ○
13-1	nonassertive ✗	assertive
14-1	assertive ✓	aggressive

15 -1	nonassertive ✗	assertive
16 -1	assertive ✓	aggressive
17 -2	nonassertive	assertive ✓
18 -3	nonassertive	assertive ✓
19 -0	nonassertive ✗	assertive
20 -1	assertive ✓	aggressive

Add up the number of questions you answered toward the assertive end of the scale. Then get the total you answered toward the other end. To profile your results, draw a line across each column below at the point that represents your score. Shade in the areas from zero to the line you have drawn in each column.

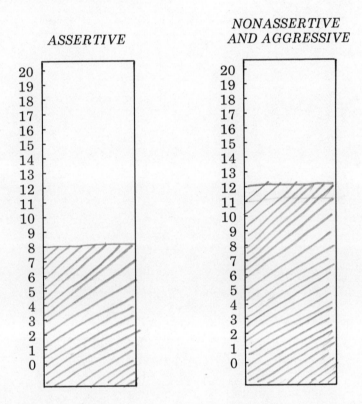

ASSERTIVE

NONASSERTIVE
AND AGGRESSIVE

DISCUSSION GUIDE

After scoring your answĕrs to the twenty questions, divide into small groups to discuss the following:

1. How do nonassertive, assertive, and aggressive behaviors relate to sex roles?

2. Which behaviors are common among nurses? Why?

3. What assertive responses can you formulate for each of the questions in which you scored at the opposite end of the scale?

4. What rights do you believe people should have in their relationships with others?

7

Hurting and Being Hurt

DIRECTIONS

In the space below write twenty sentences in which the word *hurt* is used.

1.

2.

3.

4.

5.

6.

7.

8.

9.

10.

11.

12.

13.

14.

15.

16.

17.

18.

19.

20.

DISCUSSION GUIDELINES

This exercise focuses on the expression of hurt in both the emotional and the physical sense and the ease or difficulty with which you acknowledge being hurt. It may also encourage you to become aware of specific areas of emotional vulnerability. The following questions may be helpful.

1. How often, and in what ways, did you refer to hurt in yourself as opposed to hurt in others?

2. Did you tend to use the word *hurt* in an active or a passive sense?

3. Did you tend to use the word *hurt* in an emotional or a physical sense?

4. Under what circumstances are you hurt?

5. Under what circumstances do you hurt others?

6. How do you reduce emotional hurt within yourself?

Colleague Relations Inventory

The following exercise, based on the Johari Window,* is designed to enable you to examine your own and your group's receptivity to feedback, willingness to self-disclose, and willingness to take risks in relations with each other. It uses an inventory adapted from a managerial effectiveness survey developed by Jay Hall to assess your understanding of and behavior in your interpersonal relationships. There are no right or wrong answers. The best answer is the one that comes closest to representing your own practices.

DIRECTIONS

Complete the Colleague Relations Inventory, recording your answers on the Colleague Relations Inventory Answer Sheet following (on page 27). For each item indicate which of the alternative reactions would be more characteristic of the way you would handle the situation described. Some alternatives may be equally characteristic of you or equally uncharacteristic. While this is a possibility, nevertheless choose the alternative which is *relatively* more characteristic of you. For each item, you will have five points that you may distribute in any of the following combinations:

	A	B
If A is completely characteristic of what you would do and B is completely uncharacteristic, write 5 on the answer sheet under A and 0 under B, thus:	5	0
If A is considerably characteristic of what you would do and B is somewhat characteristic, write 4 on the answer sheet under A and 1 under B, thus:	4	1

Source: David W. Johnson, REACHING OUT: Interpersonal Effectiveness and Self-Actualization, ©1972, pp. 20-25. Adapted by permission of Prentice-Hall, Inc., Englewood Cliffs, New Jersey.

*See J. Luft and H. Ingham, "The Johari Window, a Graphic Model of Awareness in Interpersonal Relations," in *Group Processes: An Introduction to Group Dynamics*, by J. Luft (Palo Alto: Calif.: National Press Books, 1963), pp. 10-12.

If A is only slightly more characteristic of
what you would do than B is, write 3 under
A and 2 under B, thus: 3   2

Each of the above three combinations may be used
in the converse order; that is, if B is slightly more
characteristic of you than A, you would write
2 under A and 3 under B. Similarly you might
write 1 under A and 4 under B or 0 under A
and 5 under B.

Thus there are six possible combinations for responding to the pair of alternatives presented
to you with each survey item. *Be sure the numbers you assign to each pair add up to 5.* In
general, try to relate each situation in the survey to your own personal experience. Take as
much time as you need to make a true and accurate response. Attempts to give a "correct"
response merely distort the meaning of your answers and render the test results valueless.

Colleague Relations Inventory

1. If a colleague of mine had a "personality conflict" with a mutual acquaintance of ours
   with whom it was important for her or him to get along, I would:

   A. Tell my colleague that I felt she or he was partially responsible for any problems
      with this other person and try to let my colleague know how the person was being
      affected by her or him.

   B. Not get involved because I wouldn't be able to continue to get along with both of
      them once I had entered in any way.

2. If one of my colleagues and I had had a heated argument in the past, and I realized
   that she or he was still not at ease around me from that time on, I would:

   A. Avoid making things worse by discussing this behavior and just let the whole thing
      drop.

   B. Bring up the behavior and ask how my colleague felt the argument had affected our
      relationship.

3. If a colleague began to avoid me and act in an aloof and withdrawing manner, I would:

   A. Tell my colleague about this behavior and suggest that she or he tell me what was on
      her or his mind.

   B. Follow that person's lead and keep our contacts brief and aloof, since that seems
      to be what she or he wants.

4. If two of my colleagues and I were talking, and one of them slipped and brought up a
   personal problem of mine that involved the other colleague but of which she or he was
   not yet aware, I would:

   A. Change the subject and signal my colleague to do the same.

   B. Tell the uninformed colleague what the other colleague was talking about and suggest
      that we go into it later.

5. If a colleague were to tell me that, in her or his opinion, I was doing things that made me less effective than I might be in social situations, I would:

    A. Ask my colleague to spell out or describe what she or he had observed and to suggest changes I might make.

    B. Resent the criticism and let my colleague know why I behave the way I do.

6. If one of my colleagues aspired to an office in our organization for which I felt this person was unqualified, and if she or he had been tentatively assigned to that position by the president of our group, I would:

    A. Not mention my misgivings to either my colleague or the president and let them handle it in their own way.

    B. Tell my colleague and the president of my misgivings and then leave the final decision up to them.

7. If I felt that one of my colleagues was being unfair to me and to other colleagues, but none of us had mentioned anything about it, I would:

    A. Ask several of these people how they perceived the situation to see if they felt this colleague was being unfair.

    B. Not ask the others how they perceived our colleague, but wait for them to bring it up with me.

8. If I were preoccupied with some personal matters and a colleague told me that I had become irritated with her or him and others and that I was jumping on people for unimportant things, I would:

    A. Tell my colleague that I was preoccupied and would probably be on edge for a while and would prefer not to be bothered.

    B. Listen to the complaints but not try to explain my actions to this person.

9. If I had heard some colleagues discussing an ugly rumor about a friend of mine, which I knew could hurt my friend, and if my friend asked me whether I knew anything about it, I would:

    A. Say I didn't know anything about it and tell my friend that no one would believe a rumor like that anyway.

    B. Tell my friend exactly what I had heard, when I had heard it, and from whom I had heard it.

10. If a colleague pointed out the fact that I had a personality conflict with another colleague with whom it was important for me to get along, I would:

    A. Consider the comments out of line and tell this colleague I didn't want to discuss the matter any further.

    B   Talk about it openly to find out how my behavior was being affected by this conflict.

11. If my relationship with a colleague had been damaged by repeated arguments on an issue of importance to us both, I would:

    A. Be cautious in my conversations with this person so the issue would not come up again to worsen our relationship.

B. Point to the problems the controversy was causing in our relationship and suggest that we discuss it until we resolved it.

12. If in a personal discussion with a colleague about her or his problems and behavior this colleague suddenly suggested we discuss my problems and behavior as well, I would:

   A. Try to keep the discussion away from me by suggesting that other, closer associates often talked to me about such matters.

   B. Welcome the opportunity to hear what this colleague felt about me and encourage such comments.

13. If a colleague of mine began to tell me about her or his hostile feelings toward another associate whom she or he felt was being unkind to others (and I agreed wholeheartedly), I would:

   A. Listen and also express my own feelings so she or he would know where I stood.

   B. Listen, but not express my own negative views and opinions, because she or he might repeat what I said in confidence.

14. If I thought an ugly rumor was being spread about me and suspected that one of my colleagues had quite likely heard it, I would:

   A. Avoid mentioning the issue and leave it to my colleague to tell me about it if she or he wanted to.

   B. Risk putting my colleague on the spot by asking directly what she or he knew about the whole thing.

15. If I had observed a colleague in social situations and thought that she or he was doing a number of things that hurt these relationships, I would:

   A. Risk being seen as a busybody and tell my colleague what I had observed and my reactions to it.

   B. Keep my opinions to myself rather than be seen as interfering in things that are none of my business.

16. If two colleagues and I were talking, and one of them inadvertently mentioned a personal problem that concerned me, but of which I knew nothing, I would:

   A. Press them both for information about the problem and their opinions about it.

   B. Leave it up to my colleagues to tell me or not tell me, letting them change the subject if they wished.

17. If a colleague seemed to be preoccupied and began to jump on me for seemingly unimportant things, becoming irritated with me and others without real cause, I would:

   A. Treat that person with kid gloves for a while, on the assumption that she or he was having some temporary personal problems that were none of my business.

   B. Try to talk to the person about it and point out how this behavior was affecting people.

18. If I had begun to dislike certain habits of an associate to the point that it was interfering with my enjoyment of the person's company, I would:

A. Say nothing to the associate directly, but let her or him know my feelings by ignoring the person whenever these annoying habits were obvious.

B. Get my feelings out in the open and clear the air so that we could continue our friendship comfortably and enjoyably.

19. In discussing social behavior with one of my more sensitive colleagues, I would:

A. Avoid mentioning that person's own flaws and weaknesses so as not to hurt her or his feelings.

B. Focus on her or his flaws and weaknesses so this colleague could improve her or his interpersonal skills.

20. If I knew I might be assigned to an important position in our group and my colleagues' attitudes toward me had become rather negative, I would:

A. Discuss my shortcomings with my colleagues so I could learn where to improve.

B. Try to figure out my shortcomings by myself so I could improve.

Colleague Relations Inventory Answer Sheet

	A	B		A	B
1.	3	2	11.	3	2
2.	2	3	12.	3	2
3.	3	2	13.	3	2
4.	2	3	14.	2	3
5.	2	3	15.	3	2
6.	3	2	16.	3	2
7.	3	2	17.	2	3
8.	2	3	18.	4	1
9.	1	4	19.	4	1
10.	1	4	20.	2	3

EXPLANATION OF SCORING

Ten of the inventory questions deal with your receptivity to feedback from colleagues and ten are concerned with your willingness to self-disclose, be open, or give feedback to your colleagues. Transfer your scores from the Inventory Answer Sheet to the Inventory Answer Key that follows. Add the scores in the Receptivity to Feedback column; then add the scores in the Willingness to Self-Disclose column. Do not enter any points for the alternatives not listed in the key (they measure neither receptivity to feedback nor willingness to self-disclose).

Colleague Relations Inventory Answer Key

RECEPTIVITY TO FEEDBACK	WILLINGNESS TO SELF-DISCLOSE
2. B _3_	1. A _3_
3. A _3_	4. B _3_
5. A _2_	6. B _2_
7. A _3_	9. B _4_
8. B _3_	11. B _2_
10. B _4_	13. A _3_
12. B _2_	15. A _3_
14. B _3_	17. B _3_
16. A _3_	18. B _1_
20. A _2_	19. B _1_
Total _28_	Total _25_

On the Colleague Relations Inventory Summary Sheet below, add the total for receptivity to feedback to the total for willingness to self-disclose to arrive at an index of interpersonal risk taking. To get the results of the inventory for the group as a whole, add the scores of every member, and divide by the number of persons in the group. Enter the group scores on the summary sheet.

Colleague Relations Inventory Summary Sheet

	YOUR SCORES	GROUP AVERAGE SCORES
Receptivity to feedback	28	
Willingness to self-disclose	25	
Interpersonal risk taking (total)		

In the boxes below, draw horizontal and vertical lines through your scores and the group's scores for receptivity to feedback and willingness to self-disclose. The results should look like the Johari Window.

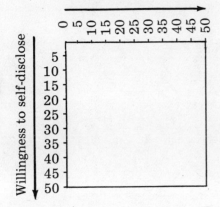

YOUR SCORES
Receptivity to feedback

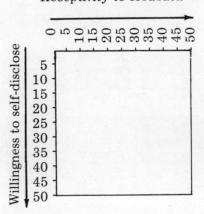

GROUP AVERAGE SCORES
Receptivity to feedback

DISCUSSION GUIDELINES

Discuss the results in the group as a whole. The following questions may facilitate your discussion:

1. What are your thoughts and feelings about the appropriate times to receive feedback from and to self-disclose to your colleagues?

2. When do you want other members of the group to give feedback to you and when do you want to self-disclose to them?

3. Is your group conservative or risky on the whole?

4. How does trust affect your receptivity to feedback and willingness to give feedback?

5. Would you like to change the way you are now behaving?

6. What changes in your behavior would be productive and useful to develop better relationships with your colleagues?

The Ten Commandments

DIRECTIONS

Use the form below to write out as many of the Ten Commandments as you can recall.

THE TEN COMMANDMENTS

Compare your list with the actual commandments below.

1. I am the Lord thy God, which have brought thee out of the land of Egypt, out of the house of bondage. Thou shalt have no other gods before me.

2. Thou shalt not make unto thee any graven image, or any likeness of any thing that is in heaven above, or that is in the earth beneath, or that is in the water under the earth. Thou shalt not bow down thyself to them, nor serve them: for I the Lord thy God am a jealous God, visiting the iniquity of the fathers upon the children unto the third and fourth generation of them that hate me; and shewing mercy unto thousands of them that love me, and keep my commandments.

3. Thou shalt not take the name of the Lord thy God in vain; for the Lord will not hold him guiltless that taketh his name in vain.

4. Remember the sabbath day, to keep it holy. Six days shalt thou labor, and do all thy work. But the seventh day is the sabbath of the Lord thy God: in it thou shalt not do any work, thou, nor thy son, nor thy daughter, thy manservant, nor thy maidservant, nor thy cattle, nor thy sojourner who is within thy gates. For in six days the Lord made heaven and earth, the sea, and all that in them is, and rested the seventh day: wherefore the Lord blessed the sabbath day, and hallowed it.

5. Honor thy father and thy mother: that thy days may be long in the land which the Lord thy God giveth thee.

6. Thou shalt not kill.

7. Thou shalt not commit adultery.

8. Thou shalt not steal.

9. Thou shalt not bear false witness against thy neighbor.

10. Thou shalt not covet thy neighbor's house, thou shalt not covet thy neighbor's wife, nor his manservant, nor his maidservant, nor his ox, nor his ass, nor any thing that is thy neighbor's.

DISCUSSION GUIDELINES

After comparing your list with the actual commandments, discuss the personal significance of your distortions of recall, your omissions, and the order in which you recalled the Ten Commandments.

Now write out ten personal commandments that you would like to be able to follow.

MY OWN TEN COMMANDMENTS

DISCUSSION GUIDELINES

Read your personal commandments aloud to the group and discuss them, considering the following questions:

1. Which commandments are unrealistic? Arbitrary? Coercive? Cliché ridden?

2. What are the relevance and value of each commandment for you?

3. Are cultural myths and shibboleths reflected in your commandments?

4. To what extent may the beliefs and values reflected in your commandments influence your therapeutic interactions with clients?

Self-Disclosure Activity

Self-disclosure is most clearly done when you tell others directly how you are reacting to the present situation. Yet many times people reveal themselves in indirect ways, for example, by the jokes they tell, the things they find funny, the books they are interested in, or the movies they see. All these actions and attitudes tell others something about a person. Often people may learn something about themselves that they were not fully aware of by analyzing their dreams, daydreams, interests, values, or humor. This exercise lets you use your imagination in ways that may lead you to a greater self-awareness and that may help each of you get to know one another in a different and interesting way.

DIRECTIONS

The following list presents fantasy situations that deal with initiating relationships with lonely people or giving help to individuals who seem to need it. Divide into groups of three. The leader will present an unfinished fantasy situation to each triad. Think about your ending to the fantasy situation. If you want to, write out your ending. Share with the others in your triad your ending to the fantasy situation.

    The fantasy situations are:

1. You are walking down the hall of a pediatric unit. From one of the rooms you hear a little girl crying. What do you do? What happens?

2. You are eating lunch in the hospital cafeteria. You get your lunch and walk into the lunchroom. The lunchroom is crowded and noisy, with lots of people laughing, shouting, and having a good time. Off in a corner is another nursing student sitting all alone at a table. What do you do? What happens?

3. You are going to a party. You enter the house, take off your coat, find something to drink, and talk to a couple of friends. Standing all by himself in the middle of the room is a man you don't know. After ten minutes the man is still standing by himself. What do you do? What happens?

Source: David W. Johnson, REACHING OUT: Interpersonal Effectiveness and Self-Actualization, © 1972, pp. 30-32. Adapted by permission of Prentice-Hall, Inc., Englewood Cliffs, New Jersey.

4. You are giving medications on a medical unit. You are talking with several of the patients in the room when a patient whom you casually met the day before walks in. He is making obnoxious and embarrassing remarks to the other patients. You walk over to him, and he insults you. What do you do? What happens?

5. You are sitting in class. Several of your classmates are making belittling comments to another student. The student is obviously feeling hurt. She catches your eye and looks at you. What do you do? What happens?

6. You are watching a group of patients talking in the dayroom of a psychiatric unit. A patient whom they consider odd and strange walks up to them and tries to join in the conversation. They ignore him. Finally one of the patients says, "Why don't you get lost." The patient turns away. What do you do? What happens?

7. You are sitting in a classroom. A student with whom you are not friendly has constantly annoyed the teacher and caused trouble since the class began several months ago. Although she is often funny, everyone is fed up with her behavior. She comes into the room and takes a seat next to you. What do you do? What happens?

8. There is a new teacher in the school. You have often heard her say that the program here is not nearly as good as at the school where she taught previously and that the students at your school are really lazy and uninteresting. What do you do?

DISCUSSION GUIDELINES

Share what you have learned about yourself and the other two members of your triad from the endings you gave to the fantasy situation. Then discuss the following questions:

1. What are the risks in being self-disclosing with another person? When is it better not to be open about your reactions to another person? Give examples.

2. What are the benefits from being self-disclosing with another person? When is it necessary, and when is it merely helpful? Give examples.

3. Does self-disclosure refer only to verbal behavior? Can a person be self-disclosing without using words?

4. What kinds of behavior can lead you to feel that you are being self-disclosing when others do not see you as self-disclosing at all?

5. Is there a difference between "telling somebody off" and being self-disclosing with a person? Is there a difference between passing judgment on another person and being self-disclosing with that person?

Switch partners and repeat the process of fantasizing and sharing your fantasy about another situation. This time, focus on the kinds of behavior that indicate that you are ready for others to share with you their reactions to your behavior and their impressions of you. In your group discuss the following questions:

1. What do the members of your group do that leads you to feel they want or do not want you to be self-disclosing with them?

2. Describe specific actions of any member that (a) make it easier to be self-disclosing with that person, or (b) make it difficult for you to be self-disclosing with that person.

3. Take no more than twenty minutes to share these impressions with your fellow group members. Then see if the group can draw some general conclusions about what helps and what hinders self-disclosure in others.

Again switch partners and repeat the exercise with a different fantasy situation. This time, in discussing the exercise with the members of your triad focus on constructive self-disclosure. It is possible to self-disclose in ways that enhance a relationship or in ways that threaten it. Explore how self-disclosures can be made constructively, using the following guidelines:

1. Name the group members whose self-disclosure you find it easiest to receive. That is, name those with whom you feel most comfortable hearing their honest reactions to something you have said or done in the group.

2. What do these group members do that leads you to be receptive to their self-disclosure about their reactions to your behavior? What do other group members do that makes you less receptive to their self-disclosures to you?

3. Take no more than thirty minutes to share these impressions with your partners. Then try to draw some conclusions about what helps and what hinders receptiveness in others.

In the group as a whole, discuss what you have learned about yourself and the other members from this exercise.

Adjective Checklist

This exercise provides an opportunity for you to disclose your view of yourself to others in a group and to receive feedback on how the others perceive you.

DIRECTIONS

Go through the list of adjectives below and circle the six adjectives you think are most descriptive of yourself.

able	caring	dependent	fair
accepting	certain	derogatory	fearful
adaptable	cheerful	determined	foolish
aggressive	clever	dignified	frank
ambitious	cold	disciplined	free
annoying	complex	docile	friendly
anxious	confident	dogged	genial
authoritative	conforming	domineering	gentle
belligerent	controlled	dreamy	giving
bitter	courageous	dutiful	greedy
bold	cranky	effervescent	gruff
brave	critical	efficient	guilty
calm	cynical	elusive	gullible
carefree	demanding	energetic	happy
careless	dependable	extroverted	hard

Source: David W. Johnson, REACHING OUT: Interpersonal Effectiveness and Self-Actualization, © 1972, pp. 28-30. Adapted by permission of Prentice-Hall, Inc., Englewood Cliffs, New Jersey.

helpful	maternal	pragmatic	sarcastic
helpless	mature	precise	satisfied
honorable	merry	pretending	scientific
hostile	modest	pretentious	searching
idealistic	mystical	principled	self-accepting
imaginative	naive	progressive	self-actualizing
immature	narcissistic	protective	self-assertive
impressionable	negative	proud	self-aware
inconsiderate	nervous	quarrelsome	self-conscious
independent	neurotic	questioning	self-effacing
ingenious	noisy	quiet	self-indulgent
innovative	normal	radical	selfish
insensitive	oblivious	rational	self-righteous
insincere	objective	rationalizing	sensible
intelligent	observant	reactionary	sensitive
introverted	obsessive	realistic	sentimental
intuitive	organized	reasonable	serious
irresponsible	original	reassuring	shy
irritable	overburdened	rebellious	silly
jealous	overconfident	reflective	simple
jovial	overconforming	regretful	sinful
juvenile	overemotional	rejecting	skillful
kind	overprotecting	relaxed	sly
knowledgeable	passive	reliable	sociable
lazy	paternal	religious	spontaneous
learned	patient	remote	stable
lewd	perceptive	resentful	strained
liberal	perfectionist	reserved	strong
lively	persuasive	resolute	stubborn
logical	petty	respectful	sympathetic
loving	playful	responsible	taciturn
malicious	pleasant	responsive	tactful
manipulative	pompous	retentive	temperamental
materialistic	powerful	rigid	tenacious

tender	uncertain	useful	wise
tense	unconcerned	vain	wishful
thoughtful	uncontrolled	vapid	withdrawn
tough	understanding	visionary	witty
trusting	unpredictable	vulnerable	worried
trustworthy	unreasonable	warm	youthful
unassuming	unstructured	willful	zestful
unaware			

DISCUSSION GUIDELINES

Divide into groups of about five. Share with the other members of your group the adjectives you circled. Receive feedback from the other members about the adjectives they would have checked to describe you. Spend only five to ten minutes on each person in the group. Then explore the agreements and disagreements in perceptions that surfaced, and consider what their sources might be.

Who's in Charge—Your Parent, Adult, or Child?

This learning activity is based on transactional analysis theory.* Three different ego states, Parent, Adult, and Child, are represented in three scales of fifteen items each.

DIRECTIONS

Look at the three sets of statements below. If you agree more than you disagree with a statement, mark a plus (+) beside it. If you disagree more than you agree, mark a minus (−). Be sure to place either a plus or a minus to the left of each number.

The Parent Scale

( ) 1. People today just don't have enough courage to stand up for what is right.

( ) 2. The effective psychiatric nurse is a strong, tough-minded sort of person.

( ) 3. Severe punishment is justified because it stops people from doing wrong.

( ) 4. If divorces were not so easy to obtain, marriages would be taken more seriously.

( ) 5. Patients are better off if they accept what the hospital staff tells them rather than adopt a questioning approach.

( ) 6. I tend to make statements that begin with "You should," "They ought," "It's never," etc.

( ) 7. Suicide is wrong.

( ) 8. I tend to want to run things or take charge.

( ) 9. Patients don't have enough respect for nurses and doctors.

( ) 10. People who are too submissive, ingratiating, or vacillating anger or disgust me.

( ) 11. Nurses should be more dedicated to certain fundamental truths about morals, right and wrong, human nature, and so on.

*See Eric Berne, *Transactional Analysis in Psychotherapy* (New York: Grove Press, 1961).

( ) 12. It's unfortunate, but no matter how hard you try, you can't change human nature.

( ) 13. Minority groups get all the breaks.

( ) 14. I believe that hospital wards function better when the head nurse enforces rules strictly.

( ) 15. I tend to blame others for what happens more than I would like to.

The Adult Scale

( ) 1. Patients to whom I've given nursing care would say I'm decisive, yet they don't seem reluctant to disagree with me.

( ) 2. Most mistakes that people make result from misunderstanding rather than carelessness.

( ) 3. I seldom if ever blush.

( ) 4. Before starting some action I tend to gather facts and form a plan.

( ) 5. I find opinions and ideas that differ from my own interesting.

( ) 6. When I was a child, my parents encouraged me to express my views.

( ) 7. I don't usually feel bored, impatient, or lonely.

( ) 8. When it seems appropriate I can express my emotions.

( ) 9. I have attended, or would like to attend, a self-awareness or growth group.

( ) 10. Patients seem to turn to me for advice, counsel, etc., more than they turn to many nurses.

( ) 11. I find that I'm more able than most people to present a calm exterior even though I am churning inside.

( ) 12. It is possible to be honest and truthful with others.

( ) 13. I seem to have little need to dominate patients, but I also seldom, if ever, feel dominated by them.

( ) 14. People are capable of sustained self-direction and control.

( ) 15. I seem to be more comfortable than many people I know with a long period of silence.

The Child Scale

( ) 1. Humor seems to be a good way to lessen the tension in situations that are too serious.

( ) 2. I find myself becoming upset when I don't get my own way.

( ) 3. Perhaps more so than others, I'm concerned when patients display their negative emotions such as anger, boredom, etc.

( ) 4. Most important life decisions are made on the basis of feelings rather than logic.

( ) 5. I'm overconcerned about the approval of others.

( ) 6. If a psychiatrist or someone with higher authority than I have assumes the responsibility for a "tough" decision that imposes a considerable hardship on some people, I'll help carry it out.

( ) 7. I seem to cry more than most people do.

( ) 8. Sometimes I catch myself laughing too loudly or talking too loudly.

( ) 9. I feel more comfortable in "structured" situations.

( ) 10. Persons in positions of higher authority often belittle their subordinates.

( ) 11. I don't understand why, but there are times when I seem to get the "short end of the stick."

( ) 12. Driving very fast is fun.

( ) 13. There are times when I've told patients or their families "I don't make the rules, I just follow them."

( ) 14. I find sticking to a diet or quitting smoking difficult.

( ) 15. Expressions such as "Gosh," "Gee," "Golly," "Wow," are quite common in my vocabulary.

EXPLANATION OF SCORING

Each scale is scored separately. Each item answered by a plus is given a raw score of 1. Minus answers are given 0. Scores for each scale can thus range from a high of 15 to a low of 0. To profile your results, add the totals for each scale and draw a line across each column below at the point that represents your score. Shade in the area between zero and the line you have drawn in each column.

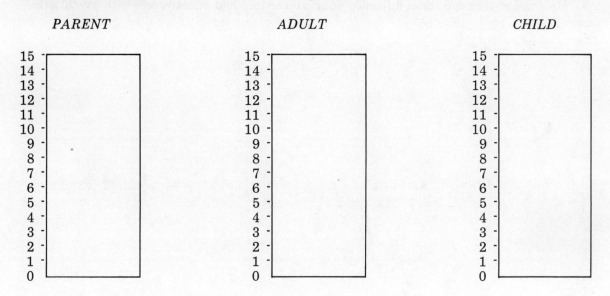

| PARENT | ADULT | CHILD |

Parent score: This represents the extent to which your behavior resembles that of a parent. This ego state is characterized by automatic use of words such as "cute," "sonny," "ought," "should," "must," "always," "disgusting," "naughty," etc. The Parent is "never wrong."

Adult score: This represents the extent to which your behavior is a function of logical processing of facts offered by the here-and-now environment. This ego state also engages in probability estimating. The Adult says, "I will."

Child score: This represents the extent to which your behavior resembles that of children. In this ego state, oaths, exclamations, name calling, and the use of such words as "gee," "I'll try," and "maybe" are typical.

Your highest raw score indicates the ego state you use most. The greater the difference between this score and your next highest score, the more dominant the ego state. The lesser the difference the more likely it is that you switch back and forth between the two ego states.

It is desirable that the Adult ego state be dominant. Most people want to increase their Adult and decrease their Parent. The Child ego state is of less concern, unless it is either too high or too low. Some typical problem profiles are:

· High Parent, low Adult, low Child (the Archie Bunker type)

· Low Parent, low Adult, high Child (Edith Bunker, Archie's wife)

DISCUSSION GUIDELINES

After you have each arrived at your total scores for each ego state, discuss the ego states by name, considering these questions:

1. What in your life experience might have led to the dominance of one ego state over another? To similarity in strength of two ego states?

2. Would you have been able to predict your ego state scores?

3. How might your ego states influence your interactions and effectiveness with psychiatric clients?

Sexual Attitude Survey

DIRECTIONS

For each of the following statements select the response that best describes your current attitude, based on the following scale:

1 Strongly agree   4 Slightly disagree

2 Agree   5 Disagree

3 Slightly agree   6 Strongly disagree

_3_ 1. Mutual masturbation by two ten-year-olds of the *same* sex is a danger signal meriting deep parental concern.

_4_ 2. Strict suppression of pornography would probably lead to a significant decrease in rape and other sex crimes.

_5_ 3. I cannot help feeling some distaste at the thought of elderly people engaging in sex.

_4_ 4. In view of the strains that population growth puts on the earth, Americans should limit their families to no more than two children.

_5_ 5. In my own marriage, I would consider it more important for the husband than the wife to be sexually experienced.

_4_ 6. Homosexuality between consenting adults is a natural and acceptable pattern of sexual response.

_4_ 7. A woman who has had premarital sexual intercourse with several partners is less likely to be satisfied with one marital partner than a man with comparable experience.

_5_ 8. It is the woman's responsibility to protect herself against pregnancy.

_6_ 9. Mate-swapping among consenting participants should be regarded as an acceptable sexual activity.

Source: Adapted from mimeographed handout, Department of Nursing, Sonoma State College, Rohnert Park, Calif., 1978.

___4___ 10. Masturbation should not be used as a release of sexual tension if a suitable sexual partner is available.

___4___ 11. A common danger of pornographic films is that the more of them one sees, the more one wants to see.

___3___ 12. Parents of adolescent children should provide them with either birth control information or names of agencies that provide such information.

___4___ 13. Regular masturbation by females before puberty may endanger the achievement of orgasm through intercourse after puberty.

___3___ 14. It is not unusual for someone to be in love with more than one person at a time.

___3___ 15. People have the right to have as many children as they can afford to raise.

___3___ 16. Religious groups should not use doctrine to prevent their members from making individual decisions about their own sexual behavior.

___3___ 17. Parents should allow their daughters as much sexual freedom as they allow their sons.

___3___ 18. It is important for sexual partners to achieve simultaneous orgasm.

___3___ 19. Having daydreams about raping someone or being raped is a danger signal of sexual maladjustment.

___6___ 20. The state should set aside beaches for nude sunbathers.

___3___ 21. Parents who are casual about nudity at home may arouse unhealthy curiosity in their children.

___4___ 22. The principal result of sex change operations is mutilation.

___5___ 23. A woman who orally stimulates her partner is performing a submissive act.

___4___ 24. Women who masturbate with a vibrator frequently become indifferent to intercourse with men.

___3___ 25. An adult who has impulsively fondled a child's genitals usually has an emotional disturbance requiring psychotherapy.

DISCUSSION GUIDELINES

In seminar or conference, compare your answers with those of others in the group. Discuss responses to specific items, considering:

1. How strongly are your beliefs held?

2. Are there themes or patterns in your responses?

3. How might your own attitudes influence your work with clients?

14

The Great Blizzard

An unrelenting blizzard of enormous proportions has virtually paralyzed a large eastern city located on one of the Great Lakes. "White-outs" caused by forty-mile-per-hour howling winds, gusting to fifty-five, have stranded anyone unfortunate enough to be away from home. Roads and highways are impassable, with drifts rising to ten feet. Smaller buildings and houses are blocked by the high drifts and by cars completely covered with snow.

The mayor and county executive have just declared a state of emergency. Meteorologists with the National Weather Service predict an unprecedented snowfall, with high winds continuing for the next seventy-two to ninety-six hours. The outdoor temperature is $10°$ F. However, the high winds have brought the chill factor to $-22°$ F. Overnight the temperature is expected to reach $0°$ F. with a $-35°$ F. wind chill factor. The metropolitan Department of Streets and Highways has declared that cleanup and removal efforts cannot even begin until the snow and winds subside.

Thirty-one people find themselves stranded in a popular restaurant and bar. Some are women and children who were out shopping and left their stranded automobiles to seek shelter from the cold and wind. Others are workers who had set out to reach their suburban homes. A few are patrons. Because there was a large political fund-raising party at the restaurant the evening before and several delivery trucks failed to arrive earlier that afternoon, many of the restaurant's food stores are depleted. Although there is a large supply of liquor, there is sufficient food for thirty-one people for only two days. Newscasters have been warning of the possibility of food, gas, electricity, and water shortages or malfunctions. Among the thirty-one marooned persons are the following eight:

Sister Mary Marcia Sutter, twenty-nine, a Catholic nun, the elected head of Religious for Ecumenical Freedom, an outspoken group of nuns and priests opposed to the conservative views of the bishop of the diocese.

Jerry ("The Fox") Rosso, forty-five, an underworld don and the owner of the Riviera, the restaurant and bar hosting the stranded travelers.

Irene Ostrander, thirty-six, chief administrator of an 800-bed general hospital and an ambitious community leader.

Dr. C. Elizabeth Byrd, forty, a clinical psychologist in private practice and a crisis consultant to community caretaker groups such as the state police and local fire department.

Jean-Jacques Krause, twenty-five, a former Olympic downhill ski racer, on his way to Blue Mountain to serve as director of the ski school and manager of Quest, its outdoor survival training program.

Louie Boles, forty-seven, a former air force career officer, now the public relations man for a United States senator.

Shirley Monroe, fifty, an attorney and a candidate for judge of the family court.

Paul Wolchyk, thirty-seven, the owner of a string of shoe stores and a small business management consultant.

DIRECTIONS

In groups of about five, take up to thirty minutes to decide which of these eight persons would emerge in a leadership role. How would the leadership come about? Why?

DISCUSSION GUIDELINES

1. What conditions in the story influenced the decisions your group made?

2. Identify the values that influenced you to select one person over another.

3. Did you place greater importance on maintaining good relationships among the stranded persons or on accomplishing the task of survival?

15

Nurse's Goals for Self

This tool can be used to help you to identify your learning goals in interactions with clients.

DIRECTIONS

In the spaces below, formulate short-term and long-term goals for yourself, and identify the plan and methods by which you intend to achieve your goals. Complete this tool a total of three times:

1. After your first session with a client (whether individual, group, or family).
2. Approximately one-third of the way through the relationship.
3. Approximately two-thirds of the way through the relationship.

Before filling out the form the first time, duplicate sufficient copies of it for each use.

SHORT-TERM GOALS	PLAN AND METHODS FOR ACHIEVING GOALS

LONG-TERM GOALS	PLAN AND METHODS FOR ACHIEVING GOALS

16

Self-Assessment Tool

Therapeutic use of self as a psychiatric nurse requires that you know yourself and your own personal needs before trying to help another person. Your unrecognized and unmet needs may interfere with your ability to be helpful.

DIRECTIONS

On the list below, rank the depth of your own personal needs, according to the following scale:

1 Minimal   4 Quite a bit

2 Little   5 Very high

3 Some

Complete this task individually, and engage in introspection.

_____ 1.	Like	_____ 10.	Be taken care of
_____ 2.	Be liked	_____ 11.	Succeed
_____ 3.	Control	_____ 12.	Be wanted
_____ 4.	Be controlled	_____ 13.	Be aggressive
_____ 5.	Love	_____ 14.	Judge
_____ 6.	Be stubborn	_____ 15.	Be judged
_____ 7.	Be accepted	_____ 16.	Seek approval
_____ 8.	Be pleasant	_____ 17.	Be included
_____ 9.	Rescue		

DISCUSSION GUIDELINES

With a peer, discuss your identification of personal needs, their depth, the life experiences that may have influenced these needs, the behaviors you generally use to see that your needs are met, and the possible effects of such needs on your interactions with clients and colleagues.

PART II

Psychiatric Nursing
Assessments

Client Assessment Form

DIRECTIONS

Using data from your process recordings, complete the following guide for assessing your client's assets and coping deficits.

FOCUS	ASSETS	PROBLEMS

A. Ability to assume responsibilities for self-care
 	
  1. Physical care
 	
    a. Personal hygiene
 	
    b. Maintenance of body functions
 	
  2. Observance of common safety measures
 	
  3. Use of manual skills		

Source: Janet A. Simmons, *The Nurse-Client Relationship in Mental Health Nursing* (Philadelphia: W. B. Saunders Co., 1976), pp. 154-57.

	FOCUS	*ASSETS*	*PROBLEMS*
	4. Use of cognitive skills		
	5. Use of skill in interpersonal relations		
	a. With relatives		
	b. With peers		
	c. With authority figures		
	d. With nurse		
B.	Accomplishment of developmental level tasks		
	1. Trust		
	2. Autonomy		
	3. Initiative		
	4. Industry		

FOCUS	ASSETS	PROBLEMS
5. Identity		
6. Intimacy		
7. Generativity		
8. Integrity		
C. Communication		
1. Accuracy		
2. Clarity		
3. Descriptive ability		
4. Preciseness		
5. Use of concrete terms		
6. Use of abstract terms		

	FOCUS	*ASSETS*	*PROBLEMS*
	7. Use of logical associations		
D.	Perception of reality 1. View of self 2. Body image 3. Interpretation of environment 4. Interpretation of others in environment		

Milieu Assessment Tool

DIRECTIONS

Using data assembled in your process recording notes, complete the following guide to assess the strengths and weaknesses of your client's milieu.

MILIEU ASPECT	*STRENGTHS*	*WEAKNESSES*
Provisions for support of physical needs		
Provisions for support of physical comfort		
Provisions for support of psychological comfort		

Source: Janet A. Simmons, *The Nurse-Client Relationship in Mental Health Nursing* (Philadelphia: W. B. Saunders Co., 1976), pp. 162-63.

MILIEU ASPECT	STRENGTHS	WEAKNESSES
Provisions for support of sociocultural needs (affiliation etc.)		
Personal space		
Personal time		
Possibility of change		
Greatest asset		
Greatest weakness		

Neurological Assessment Form

DIRECTIONS

Based on data collected through observation of a client, complete the neurological assessment form using the codes explained below.

TIME & DATE	*PUPILS*			*L.O.C.*	*S-R*	*T.R.*	*MOTOR*				*TOTAL*
	R	*< = >*	*L*				*RUE*	*RLE*	*LUE*	*LLE*	*MAX. 25*

EXPLANATION OF CODES

Pupils

Reaction time, right (R) and left (L)

(2) Reacts briskly

Source: Karen Bolin, "Assessing the Status of Neurological Patients." Copyright 1977, American Journal of Nursing Company. Reproduced with permission from American Journal of Nursing, September, vol. 77, no. 9, pp. 1478-79.

(1)   Reacts slowly

(0)   No reaction

Size

(=)   Equal

(<)   Right lesser than left

(>)   Right greater than left

Level of Consciousness (L.O.C.)

(5)   Alert and oriented x 3 = awakens easily; oriented to person, place, time

(4)   Alert and partially oriented = awakens easily but oriented in only one or two of the three spheres

(3)   Lethargic but oriented = slow to arouse, possibly slurred speech, but oriented x 3

(2)   Lethargic and disoriented = slow to arouse, oriented in only one or two spheres or completely disoriented

OR

(2)   Restless/combative (confused) = spontaneously thrashing about in bed; striking out at others; inattentive to commands

(1)   Responds to stimulation only = exhibits only some type of withdrawal or posturing in response to stimulation

(0)   Unresponsive = gives no response of any kind

Stimulus-Response (S-R)

(5)   Responds to commands = gives appropriate responses to orientation questions, complies with instructions on hand grasp, toe wiggling, etc.

(4)   Responds to name = opens eyes to name or gives some indication that he or she hears (nods, moves, etc.), but does not follow all commands

(3)   Responds to shaking = responds only to vigorous physical stimulation

(2)   Responds to pinprick = responds to light pain applied with pin to trunk or extremities to elicit either withdrawal or posturing

(1)   Responds to deep pain = responds only to mandibular pressure, periorbital rub, sternal rub, or pinch

(0)   Unresponsive = gives no response to any stimulus

Type of Response (T.R.)

(3)   Complex withdrawal = withdrawal and attempt to remove stimulus

(2) Simple withdrawal = withdrawal from stimulus alone

(1) Posturing = decorticate—head, arms, and hands flexed; decerebrate—head extended, arms extended and pronated, back arched

(0) Flaccid = no response

Motor

Right Upper Extremity (RUE)

Right Lower Extremity (RLE)

Left Upper Extremity (LUE)

Left Lower Extremity (LLE)

(2) Full spontaneous use = moves designated extremity or extremities with or *without* any stimulus

(1) Moves to stimulus only = responds only to touch, pin, or deep pain

(0) No movement = does not respond to any stimulus

Weakness of an extremity is indicated by writing "weaker" under the appropriate column.

Diagraming Interactions in in Milieus

The simplest technique for studying the social structure of a hospital unit milieu is to use diagrams such as figure 1 (next page). A major purpose of assessing a milieu this way is to help the client take advantage of the therapeutic possibilities on a psychiatric unit. In order to promote healthy socialization, staff members first need to study the unit's existing social structure.

People often become psychiatric clients because they have not learned to live comfortably in social relationships with others. They need experience in effective social living, and, in many hospitals, the psychiatric unit has become the therapeutic community that furnishes this experience. Nurses, aides, and attendants, who, in effect, live with the clients, must use the everyday experiences of the clients' lives on the unit—eating, getting up and going to sleep, meeting personal hygiene needs, working, talking, and playing together—as therapy. This is therapy with twenty-four-hour-a-day possibilities. The unit must become a setting in which there is consideration for each person's needs, where there is acceptance, understanding, and the opportunity for emotional growth.

As a nurse, you need to be constantly aware of the social relationships on the unit and the part you can play in helping the clients to improve them.

DIRECTIONS

To study the social structure of your unit, make a series of diagrams of interactions you observe at different times and places on the unit, and answer questions such as the following:

1. Who is the leader? Are there two leaders? Is there a hostile leader?

2. Who belongs to each existing group?

3. Who are the fringe members?

4. Who are the isolates?

Source: Joyce Samhammer Hays, "The Psychiatric Nurse as Sociotherapist." Copyright 1962, American Journal of Nursing Company. Reproduced with permission from American Journal of Nursing, January, vol. 62, no. 6, pp. 64-67.

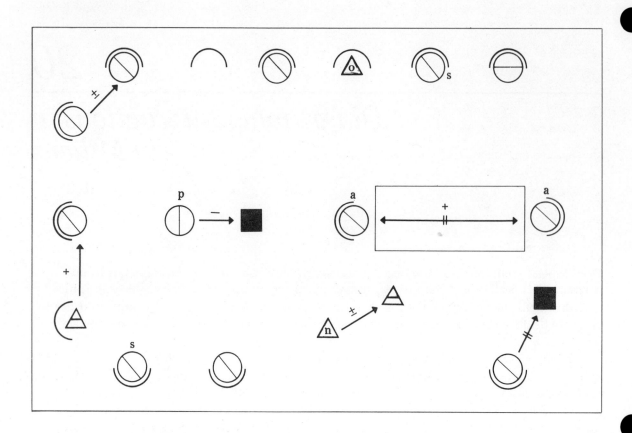

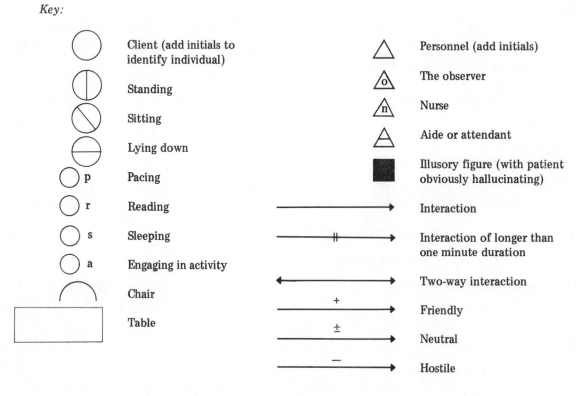

Key:

○ Client (add initials to identify individual)

⊘ Standing

⊘ Sitting

⊖ Lying down

○ p Pacing

○ r Reading

○ s Sleeping

○ a Engaging in activity

⌒ Chair

▭ Table

△ Personnel (add initials)

△ο The observer

△n Nurse

△ Aide or attendant

■ Illusory figure (with patient obviously hallucinating)

———→ Interaction

——‖—→ Interaction of longer than one minute duration

←———→ Two-way interaction

——+—→ Friendly

——±—→ Neutral

——−—→ Hostile

Figure 1. Sample interaction diagram of an inpatient milieu

5. Where does the most socializing occur: in the dining room, dayrooms, occupational therapy, outdoors, etc.?

6. Is there competition among the clients to be the "sickest"?

7. What persons or what activities promote friendly interaction?

8. What persons or activities block friendly interaction?

9. With which patients do personnel spend most time and effort?

10. What clients need individual help before they can interact independently with others and become a part of the unit society?

11. What opportunities are there to foster competence in group living—client government, remotivation groups, discussion groups, activity groups? Can you handle discussions on such topics as family relationships, managing angry feelings, making friends, working and competing with others, attitudes, and authority figures? Can you help each client to think "we" instead of "I"?

USING INTERACTION DIAGRAMS

Diagraming can be of inestimable value in helping you to answer these questions. It is of particular value when a new client is introduced, and the therapeutic team wishes to study the newcomer's manner of relating to or withdrawing from the group and the role he or she plays in the unit. Diagraming can help you to capitalize on client "clusters"—it may reveal clients who exclude themselves or are excluded. However, a single diagram made at one particular time has little significance. Only when you have made many diagrams at different times of day, on different days, and in different places over a period of time, can you draw valid conclusions about recurring patterns.

The interaction diagram can be used by all levels of nursing personnel. As you continue to use it and discuss the findings it reveals with other personnel, you will all become acutely aware of those clients who need the most help in interacting with others. Clients who have the greatest problems in interacting, because they either withdraw or relate in a hostile fashion, can be selected for more intensive individual nurse-client relationships. Personnel who avoid relating to clients or who relate nontherapeutically can be counseled. Client leadership potential can be discovered and encouraged. You can evaluate objectively which activities promote friendly interaction and which ones hinder it. Clients can learn the technique of diagraming and can chart their group progress from social disorganization to social integration. The unit milieu is not static but dynamic and changing. Only if you keep aware of this factor can you introduce constructive changes.

Observation of Nonverbal Behavior

DIRECTIONS

From your observations of a client, select an example of nonverbal behavior. Describe it on the form provided below.

Client's nonverbal behavior	
Meaning of behavior	
Assessment of apparent reasons for behavior	

Nursing intervention	
Outcome of intervention	
Evaluation of effectiveness of intervention	
Suggested alternative intervention	

Life Crises Scale

Researchers Holmes and Masuda have concluded that clusters of certain life events help to make a person vulnerable to illness. They found that the events of ordinary life—such as marriage, vacation, a new job—can help to trigger illness because they require energy to cope with them and therefore reduce a person's resistance to illness.

DIRECTIONS

Using yourself or a client as the subject, place a check mark on the line to the left of each event that has occurred in the subject's life during the past year. If the event has occurred more than once, place a check mark for each occurrence.

____ 1. Death of spouse	____ 13. Sexual difficulties
____ 2. Divorce	✓ 14. Gain of new family member
____ 3. Marital separation	____ 15. Business readjustment
____ 4. Jail term	✓ 16. Change in financial state
____ 5. Death of close family member	____ 17. Death of close friend
____ 6. Personal injury or illness	✓ 18. Change to different line of work
____ 7. Marriage	____ 19. Change in number of arguments with spouse
____ 8. Firing from work	____
____ 9. Marital reconciliation	____ 20. Mortgage over $10,000
____ 10. Retirement	____ 21. Foreclosure of mortgage or loan
✓ 11. Change in health of family member	✓ 22. Change in responsibilities at work
____ 12. Pregnancy	____ 23. Son or daughter leaving home

Source: Adapted from Thomas H. Holmes and Minoru Masuda, "Psychosomatic Syndrome," *Psychology Today*, April 1972, p. 71. REPRINTED FROM PSYCHOLOGY TODAY MAGAZINE. Copyright ©1972 Ziff-Davis Publishing Company.

✓ 24. Trouble with in-laws

___ 25. Outstanding personal achievement

✓ 26. Spouse beginning or stopping work

✓ 27. Beginning or ending school

___ 28. Change in living conditions

✓ 29. Revision of personal habits

___ 30. Trouble with boss

✓ 31. Change in work hours or conditions

___ 32. Change in residence

___ 33. Change in schools

___ 34. Change in recreation

✓ 35. Change in church activities

✓ 36. Change in social activities

___ 37. Mortgage or loan less than $10,000

✓ 38. Change in sleeping habits

___ 39. Change in number of family get-togethers

___ 40. Change in eating habits

✓ 41. Vacation

✓ 42. Christmas

___ 43. Minor violations of the law

EXPLANATION OF SCORING

In the blanks to the right below, enter the listed mean value for each life event you have checked, and add up the values to get the subject's total score.

Event	Mean Value	
1	100	___
2	73	___
3	65	___
4	63	___
5	63	___
6	53	___
7	50	___
8	47	___
9	45	___
10	45	___
11	44	44
12	40	___
13	39	___
14	39	39
15	39	___
16	38	38
17	37	___
18	36	36

Event	Mean Value	
19	35	————
20	31	————
21	30	————
22	29	29
23	29	————
24	29	29
25	28	————
26	26	26
27	26	26
28	25	————
29	24	24
30	23	————
31	20	20
32	20	————
33	20	————
34	19	————
35	19	19
36	18	18
37	17	————
38	16	16
39	15	————
40	15	13
41	13	12
42	12	————
43	11	————

Subject's total ————————

Find the subject's life crises level among the following categories:

150-199	Mild risk
200-299	Moderate risk
300 or more	Major risk

The higher the risk level, the more likely it is that the subject will encounter illness within the year. Of the subjects Holmes and Masuda studied, 37 percent in the mild risk category, 51 percent in the moderate risk category, and 79 percent in the major risk category had associated health changes.

DISCUSSION GUIDELINES

In seminar or small groups, discuss these questions:

1. What are the implications of this exercise for primary prevention? Secondary prevention? Tertiary prevention?

2. What nursing actions are possible in relation to persons in the mild risk category? The moderate risk category? The major risk category?

3. Recent research indicates that the event itself (change in health of family member), and not the valence of the event (change for the better, or change for the worse), constitutes a stressful life event because it requires adaptive or coping behavior. What are the implications of this finding?

Myths about Suicide

DIRECTIONS

Mark T for true or F for false on the line to the left of each of the following statements.

_F_ 1. Women attempt suicide more often than men.

_F_ 2. Only cowards and weaklings consider suicide as an alternative.

_F_ 3. Once suicidal, always suicidal.

_F_ 4. Unfortunately, suicide happens without warning.

_F_ 5. It is better to discuss hopeful and pleasant things with a suicidal person than it is to discuss the person's suicidal intent.

_F_ 6. Suicide attempts are manipulative ploys.

_F_ 7. The surest way to commit suicide is to turn on the gas.

_F_ 8. Tendencies toward suicide are inherited.

_F_ 9. More rich people than poor people attempt suicide.

_F_ 10. Only psychotic persons try to kill themselves.

_F_ 11. If a person talks about intending to commit suicide, he or she won't do it.

_F_ 12. Suicidal persons are usually intent on dying.

_F_ 13. Suicide is seldom attempted by intelligent persons.

_F_ 14. Suicide is seldom attempted by well-educated persons.

_F_ 15. The immediate suicide risk is over when improvement follows a suicidal crisis.

EXPLANATION OF SCORING

All of the statements are *false*. These fifteen items constitute the most frequently held myths or "old wives' tales" about suicide and suicidal persons.

DISCUSSION GUIDELINES

On a chalkboard, tabulate the responses of all the students to each question. Discuss each myth in turn, considering factors such as:

1. What in your life experience might have led you to respond as you did?

2. How might your beliefs about suicide influence your interactions and effectiveness with suicidal persons?

Group Member Selection Interview Guide

DIRECTIONS

Complete this profile for each individual you interview who is a candidate for your therapy group. Before filling out the form the first time, duplicate sufficient copies of it for each use.

Potential Group Member Profile

Name: _____   Date of interview: _____

Age: _____   Length of interview: _____

Sex: _____

The problem as the client views it:

Behavioral descriptive data:

Expected effect of this client on other members:

Risk of client's premature termination:

Check yes or no for each item.	YES	NO
1. Denial is high		
2. Somatization is high		
3. Motivation is low		
4. Psychological-mindedness is low		
5. Physical reasons interfere (transportation, distance, scheduling conflict, etc.)		
6. Current life stress is high		
7. Client has problems with intimacy or disclosure		

Risk of premature termination from the group is determined by the number of items checked in the yes column. The more items checked yes, the greater the risk.

Recommendations for group therapy (including rationale):

_____

Group Leader(s)

DISCUSSION GUIDELINES

With your cotherapist or instructor, discuss the following questions:

1. What are your selection criteria for including a client within the group?

2. What are your impressions of each individual's motivation toward group treatment?

3. Considering your recommendations about membership for all candidates, what is the composition and balance of the group? What characteristics does the group have?

4. Based on your answers to question 3, what are your expectations about the possible initial behavior of the group as a whole and of its individual members?

Therapeutic Goals for Group Members

DIRECTIONS

In the form below, formulate short-term and long-term goals for each group member. Identify the approaches, interventions, or behavior you intend to use to facilitate meeting the goals. Complete this tool a total of three times:

1. After the selection interview and first group session.
2. Approximately one-third of the way through the life of the group.
3. Approximately two-thirds of the way through the life of the group.

Before filling out the form the first time, duplicate sufficient copies of it for each use.

GROUP MEMBER:		
SHORT-TERM GOALS	RATIONALE	APPROACHES
LONG-TERM GOALS	RATIONALE	APPROACHES

GROUP MEMBER:		
SHORT-TERM GOALS	RATIONALE	APPROACHES
LONG-TERM GOALS	RATIONALE	APPROACHES

GROUP MEMBER:		
SHORT-TERM GOALS	RATIONALE	APPROACHES
LONG-TERM GOALS	RATIONALE	APPROACHES

GROUP MEMBER:

SHORT-TERM GOALS	RATIONALE	APPROACHES

LONG-TERM GOALS	RATIONALE	APPROACHES

GROUP MEMBER:

SHORT-TERM GOALS	RATIONALE	APPROACHES

LONG-TERM GOALS	RATIONALE	APPROACHES

GROUP MEMBER:		
SHORT-TERM GOALS	RATIONALE	APPROACHES
LONG-TERM GOALS	RATIONALE	APPROACHES

GROUP MEMBER:		
SHORT-TERM GOALS	RATIONALE	APPROACHES
LONG-TERM GOALS	RATIONALE	APPROACHES

GROUP MEMBER:		
SHORT-TERM GOALS	RATIONALE	APPROACHES
LONG-TERM GOALS	RATIONALE	APPROACHES

GROUP MEMBER:		
SHORT-TERM GOALS	RATIONALE	APPROACHES
LONG-TERM GOALS	RATIONALE	APPROACHES

26

Assessing Group Power and Intimacy Concerns

DIRECTIONS

This tool is based on the work of Bennis and Shepard.* It may be used to analyze a group you are leading or another therapist's group. It can also be used for nontherapy groups.

1. After reviewing your data on your therapy group, complete this tool a total of four times.

   a. After one of the first five group sessions.

   b. After one of the last five sessions.

   c. After any other two sessions during the life of the group.

   Before filling out the form the first time, duplicate sufficient copies of it for each use.

2. In column 1, list the group members' names.

3. If you believe the group to be in Phase I, where concerns center around dependence and power, identify each member in column 2 as either dependent, counterdependent, or independent.

4. In column 3, identify the quality and quantity of each group member's movement toward resolution of the dependence-power struggles within the group.

5. If you believe the group to be in Phase II, where the concerns center around interdependence and intimacy, identify each member in column 4 as either overpersonal, counterpersonal, or independent.

6. In column 5, identify the quality and quantity of the group member's movement toward resolution of the interdependence-intimacy struggles within the group.

7. Answer the questions that follow the tool.

*See W. Bennis and H. A. Shepard, "A Theory of Group Development," *Human Relations* 9 (1956): 415-37.

1 GROUP MEMBER	2 PHASE I: DEPENDENCE-POWER RELATIONS	3 MOVEMENT TOWARD RESOLUTION	4 PHASE II: INTERDEPENDENCE-PERSONAL RELATIONS	5 MOVEMENT TOWARD RESOLUTION

QUESTIONS

1. What is the basis for your decision about the current group phase?

2. Identify group members who serve as "catalysts" and occurrences that served as "barometric events" in the movement toward resolution.

3. Identify therapist interventions that facilitated or hindered movement toward resolution. State the rationale for each intervention.

4. Identify future or alternative therapist interventions to aid movement toward resolution. State the rationale for each.

27

Identifying Group Inclusion Needs

This tool is based on the work of Schutz.* It may be used to analyze a group you are leading or another therapist's group. It can also be used for nontherapy groups.

DIRECTIONS

In the form below, write the group members' names in the first column. Tabulate the number of times each group member moved in either a verbal or a nonverbal way to be included. Tabulate the number of times each group member received a therapist response to this movement. Also tabulate the number of times each group member moved in either a verbal or a nonverbal way to include another. Tabulate the number of times each group member received a therapist response to this. Complete this tool a total of three times:

1. For one of the first three sessions.

2. For one of the middle sessions.

3. For one of the final three sessions.

Before filling out the form the first time, duplicate sufficient copies of it for each use.

*See W. C. Schutz, The Interpersonal Underworld: FIRO (Palo Alto, Calif.: Science and Behavior Books, 1958).

| GROUP MEMBERS | BIDS TO INCLUDE SELF | | THERAPIST RESPONSES |
	VERBAL	NONVERBAL	

| GROUP MEMBERS | BIDS TO INCLUDE OTHERS | | THERAPIST RESPONSES |
	VERBAL	NONVERBAL	

Assessing Group Inclusion Needs

This tool is based on the work of Schutz.* It may be used to analyze a group you are leading or another therapist's group. It can also be used for nontherapy groups.

DIRECTIONS

In the form below, give verbatim data from a group therapy session that demonstrates group members' inclusion needs and the therapist's responses. Analyze the data in the last column. Then answer the questions that follow the form. Complete this tool a total of three times:

1. For one of the first three sessions.

2. For one of the middle sessions.

3. For one of the final three sessions.

Before filling out the form the first time, duplicate sufficient copies of it for each use.

*See W. C. Schutz, *The Interpersonal Underworld: FIRO* (Palo Alto, Calif.: Science and Behavior Books, 1958).

VERBATIM EXAMPLE	INTERVENTION AND RATIONALE	ANALYSIS

QUESTIONS

1. Comment on the inclusion needs of the group members whose verbal and nonverbal behaviors are not included in the verbatim example column.

2. Comment on the inclusion needs of the therapist and their manifestation during this session.

3. What do these data tell you about the stage of the group?

4. Based on the preceding data and the therapist's method of dealing with the inclusion needs, what is your prediction about the future manifestation of inclusion needs within the group?

Identifying Group Control Needs

This tool is based on the work of Schutz.* It may be used to analyze a group you are leading or another therapist's group. It can also be used for nontherapy groups.

DIRECTIONS

In the form below, write the group members' names in the first column. Tabulate the number of times each group member moved in either a verbal or a nonverbal way to be controlled. Tabulate the number of times each group member received a therapist response to this bid. Also tabulate the number of times each group member moved in either a verbal or a nonverbal way to control another. Tabulate the number of times each group member received a therapist response to this. Complete this tool a total of three times:

1. For one of the first three sessions.

2. For one of the middle sessions.

3. For one of the final three sessions.

Before filling out the form the first time, duplicate sufficient copies of it for each use.

*See W. C. Schutz, *The Interpersonal Underworld: FIRO* (Palo Alto, Calif.: Science and Behavior Books, 1958).

GROUP MEMBERS	BIDS FOR CONTROL OF SELF		THERAPIST RESPONSES
	VERBAL	NONVERBAL	

GROUP MEMBERS	BIDS TO CONTROL OTHERS		THERAPIST RESPONSES
	VERBAL	NONVERBAL	

Assessing Group Control Needs

This tool is based on the work of Schutz.* It may be used to analyze a group you are leading or another therapist's group. It can also be used for nontherapy groups.

DIRECTIONS

In the form below, give verbatim data from a group session that demonstrates group members' control needs and the therapist's responses. Analyze the data in the last column. Then answer the questions that follow the form. Complete this tool a total of three times:

1. For one of the first three sessions.

2. For one of the middle sessions.

3. For one of the final three sessions.

Before filling out the form the first time, duplicate sufficient copies of it for each use.

*See W. C. Schutz, *The Interpersonal Underworld: FIRO* (Palo Alto, Calif.: Science and Behavior Books, 1958).

VERBATIM EXAMPLE	INTERVENTION AND RATIONALE	ANALYSIS

QUESTIONS

1. Comment on the control needs of the group members whose verbal and nonverbal behaviors were not included in the verbatim example column.

2. Comment on the control needs of the therapist and their manifestation during this session.

3. What do these data tell you about the stage of the group?

4. Based on the preceding data and the therapist's method of dealing with the control needs of the group, what is your prediction about the future manifestation of control needs within the group?

Identifying Group Affection Needs

This tool is based on the work of Schutz.* It may be used to analyze a group you are leading or another therapist's group. It can also be used for nontherapy groups.

DIRECTIONS

In the form below, write the group members' names in the first column. Tabulate the number of times each group member moved in either a verbal or a nonverbal way to seek affection. Tabulate the number of times each group member received a therapist response to this bid. Also tabulate the number of times each group member moved in either a verbal or a nonverbal way to give affection to another. Tabulate the number of times each group member received a therapist response to this. Complete this tool a total of three times:

1. For one of the first three sessions.

2. For one of the middle sessions.

3. For one of the final three sessions.

Before filling out the form the first time, duplicate sufficient copies of it for each use.

*See W. C. Schutz, *The Interpersonal Underworld: FIRO* (Palo Alto, Calif.: Science and Behavior Books, 1958).

GROUP MEMBERS	BIDS FOR AFFECTION		THERAPIST RESPONSES
	VERBAL	NONVERBAL	

GROUP MEMBERS	BIDS TO GIVE AFFECTION		THERAPIST RESPONSES
	VERBAL	NONVERBAL	

Assessing Group Affection Needs

This tool is based on the work of Schutz.* It may be used to analyze a group you are leading or another therapist's group. It can also be used for nontherapy groups.

DIRECTIONS

In the form below, give verbatim data from a group therapy session that demonstrates group members' affection needs and the therapist's responses. Analyze the data in the last column. Then answer the questions that follow the form. Complete this tool a total of three times:

1. For one of the first three sessions.

2. For one of the middle sessions.

3. For one of the final three sessions.

Before filling out the form the first time, duplicate sufficient copies of it for each use.

*See W. C. Schutz, *The Interpersonal Underworld: FIRO* (Palo Alto, Calif.: Science and Behavior Books, 1958).

VERBATIM EXAMPLE	INTERVENTION AND RATIONALE	ANALYSIS

QUESTIONS

1. Comment on the affection needs of the group members whose verbal and nonverbal behaviors have not been included in the verbatim example column.

2. Comment on the affection needs of the therapist and their manifestation during this session.

3. What do these data tell you about the stage of the group?

4. Based on the preceding data and the therapist's method of dealing with the affection needs, what is your prediction about the future manifestation of affection needs within the group?

Mental Health Services in Your Community

DIRECTIONS

Using the charts below, identify the mental health services, facilities, and programs available in your community, and evaluate them, using the following code:

A = Adequate

L = Limited

I = Inadequate

Community facilities for mental health treatment:

SERVICE	*AGENCY*	*ADMISSION WAITING TIME (WEEKS)*	*ASSESSMENT (A) (L) (I)*
Emergency services			
Short-term care			
Day care			
Night care			
Halfway houses			

SERVICE	AGENCY	ADMISSION WAITING TIME (WEEKS)	ASSESSMENT (A) (L) (I)
Domiciliary care			
Suicide prevention			
Crisis or walk-in clinics			
Outpatient clinics			
Home follow-ups			
Sheltered workshops			
Foster care			
Patient clubs			
Prehospital screening			
Industrial mental health services			
Consultation services			
Preventive services			
Other			

Other groups and agencies having mental health programs:

GROUP	SPECIFIC PROGRAMS	ASSESSMENT (A) (L) (I)
Clergy		
Courts		
Police		
Schools		
Welfare		
Other		

Alcoholism and Drug Addiction Services in Your Community

DIRECTIONS

Using the charts below, identify the alcoholism and drug addiction services and programs available in your community, and evaluate them, using the following code:

A = Adequate

L = Limited

I = Inadequate

Agencies providing alcoholism services and programs:

SERVICE	*AGENCY*	*ASSESSMENT* *(A) (L) (I)*
Education		
Counseling		
Case finding		
Inpatient treatment		
Aftercare		

SERVICE	AGENCY	ASSESSMENT (A) (L) (I)
Rehabilitation		
Employment		
Home follow-up		
Outpatient clinics		
Alcoholics Anonymous groups		
Family counseling		
Halfway houses		
Other		

Agencies providing drug addiction services and programs:

SERVICE	AGENCY	ASSESSMENT (A) (L) (I)
Education		
Counseling		
Case finding		
Inpatient treatment		

SERVICE	AGENCY	ASSESSMENT (A) (L) (I)
Aftercare		
Rehabilitation		
Employment		
Home follow-up		
Outpatient clinics		
Residential programs		
Family counseling		
Halfway houses		
Other		

35

Mental Retardation Services in Your Community

DIRECTIONS

Using the chart below, identify the services and programs available for the mentally retarded in your community, and evaluate them, using the following code:

A = Adequate

L = Limited

I = Inadequate

Agencies providing services and programs for mentally retarded persons:

SERVICE	AGENCY	ASSESSMENT (A) (L) (I)
Day care		
Diagnostic services		
Domiciliary services		
Foster home placement		
Public school programs		

SERVICE	AGENCY	ASSESSMENT (A) (L) (I)
Recreation		
Rehabilitation		
Sheltered workshops		
Homemaker services		
Summer camps (day)		
Summer camps (residential)		
Job placement		
Vocational training		
Parent counseling		
Home visit programs		
Nursery classes		
Mental health counseling		
Other		

PART III

Psychiatric Nursing Strategies and Skills

36

Communication Role Playing in Simulated Interviews

DIRECTIONS

In the following sample interview situations you may practice your communication skills. Divide into dyads. One of you will take the role of the client and the other the role of the nurse. Devote five minutes to the role play and ten minutes to discussion with your partner about the quality of communication that took place. Videotaping and replay, if feasible, provides an additional source of feedback.

Sample Interview Situations

1. You are making a home visit to a single, sixty-eight-year-old man, who is recuperating from a leg ulcer. He sells newspapers on a busy street corner in New York City and lives alone on a very low budget. As you sit and talk with him about how things are going, he asks you very hesitantly when he'll be able to return to work.

2. You are visiting a twenty-five-year-old, single woman who is recuperating from arm surgery. She tells you that she recently applied for a job as a teacher. The administrator doing the hiring told her that her record was excellent but, since she was about to be married, he felt he should offer the job to an equally well qualified applicant. She would no doubt want a family, he said, and he did not feel that she would be able to make the necessary commitment to the job. She says all this in a very matter-of-fact way.

3. You are working in a health screening clinic for older adults. As you are taking one client's medical history, he tells you that he is unable to satisfy his wife sexually any more. He is sixty-two years of age.

4. You are visiting a young couple, Mr. and Mrs. W, who will be having their first baby in about two weeks. You have been visiting them regularly for six months. As they talk about their plans for the time after the baby's arrival, Mr. W says that he'll be glad "when this is all over, so everyone can get back to normal."

Source: Adapted from simulated situations developed by the faculty for students in community health nursing course, Department of Nursing, Sonoma State College, Rohnert Park, Calif., 1977.

5. You are visiting a seventy-two-year-old black man, Mr. L, who lives with his wife in a second story apartment in a ghetto. He has hypertension and has recently returned home from the hospital, where he was treated for a mild stroke that left his arm weak. As you talk, you notice approximately fifteen different prescription medications on the kitchen counter. He says that he feels fine but that his wife is worried about his "blood." Mr. L looks worried, fidgets, and seems to have been drinking.

6. A severely depressed, divorced woman of fifty has been referred to you because her family is concerned about her. They report that she is "not eating" and "has been very irritable since she lost her job at the probation department." She also keeps telling the daughter with whom she lives that she does not want to be a burden. During the visit she is unable to maintain eye contact and insists that "everything will be all right soon."

7. You are visiting a twenty-year-old pregnant woman (in her second trimester) who lives in a college dorm. She says she is looking forward to the birth of the baby but casually mentions that her cousin had a baby with only three fingers on its right hand.

8. You are visiting a Mexican-American woman who is pregnant for the first time at the age of forty-five. She and her husband have waited for this baby for a long time. Both of them have lived in the United States since they left Mexico six years ago. Her husband has a job in a local restaurant.

9. Mr. H has recently been diagnosed as diabetic at age forty-two. He has been hospitalized for two weeks to "control" his diabetes and is now home. You are making a home visit to assess Mr. H's level of knowledge, cooking facilities and/or plans for maintaining his diabetic diet, and insulin regimen. Other than telling you that he has accepted his condition and does not anticipate any changes in his life-style, he has not mentioned his diabetes. You have the distinct impression that he is really quite worried about how he is going to manage.

10. You are visiting Mrs. Y, a new mother who has been trying to breast-feed her baby. The baby cries a lot, and Mrs. Y is worried that the baby might not be getting enough to eat. The doctor has told her to supplement breast-feeding with formula. Her own mother agrees with the doctor and is pressuring Mrs. Y to "give this thing up."

11. Greg, who is seventeen, was doing well in high school until about four weeks before graduation. He has been to see you, the school nurse, with several minor complaints. His parents can't understand why he is so moody and quiet lately.

DISCUSSION GUIDELINES

In your dyad, or in the group as a whole, consider the following questions:

1. How did you use principles of effective communication in the interviews?

2. What constituted the major stalls or blocks in your interviews?

3. What feedback can your partner offer about your approach to interviewing?

Black American Culture Dictionary

DIRECTIONS

Try to match each word or phrase in column A with a meaning from column B. Place the number from column B on the line provided in column A. The purpose of this tool is to test whether you share meanings with a particular culture group. The completely matched lists comprise a dictionary representative of contemporary black American vocabulary.

COLUMN A	COLUMN B
___ 1. Ax	1. Sleep
___ 2. Baby	2. I got beaten
___ 3. Bag (that's my bag)	3. Got taken
___ 4. Blade	4. Musical instrument
___ 5. Blow some jams	5. Fistfight
___ 6. Bombed out	6. Select group; finest in every way; woman
___ 7. Boo-pot	7. Eat
___ 8. Boss	8. Find out your secrets
___ 9. Bread	9. Suit
___ 10. Busted	10. Money
___ 11. Check out	11. Profession (what I do well)
___ 12. Choice	12. Money
___ 13. Close-knuckle drill	13. Be genuine
___ 14. Close that razor	14. Give him a piece of your mind
___ 15. Come outa your act	15. Listen to this; approve of something; understand

Source: From HUMAN COMMUNICATION: AN INTERPERSONAL PERSPECTIVE, by Stewart L. Tubbs and Sylvia Moss. Copyright ©1974 by Random House, Inc. Reprinted by permission of the publisher.

COLUMN A	COLUMN B
_____ 16. Cooker	16. In jail; caught
_____ 17. Cop	17. Unbelievable
_____ 18. Cop a nod	18. High from drinking
_____ 19. Cop out	19. Wind (the)
_____ 20. Cut him up	20. Stop acting silly or stupid
_____ 21. Cut me loose	21. Good-looking woman
_____ 22. Devil	22. Knife
_____ 23. Dig	23. Really fine
_____ 24. Doing a bill	24. Handgun
_____ 25. Doing a bit	25. Movie; television
_____ 26. Dough	26. I understand
_____ 27. Dropping beans	27. Good
_____ 28. Dust	28. Double-talk
_____ 29. Flaky	29. Friend
_____ 30. Flick	30. Leave me alone
_____ 31. Fox	31. Marijuana
_____ 32. Freeze	32. Home
_____ 33. From the git go	33. Date; job
_____ 34. Front	34. Taking pills to get high
_____ 35. Funny changes	35. Let's leave
_____ 36. Get yourself together	36. Square
_____ 37. Getting oiled	37. Pick at or nag
_____ 38. Gig	38. Caught by the police; fired
_____ 39. Grease	39. Drunk
_____ 40. Grip	40. Play some records
_____ 41. Hawk (the)	41. Car
_____ 42. Heavy	42. Beginning
_____ 43. Hit on the broad	43. Dope habit; hooked
_____ 44. Hog	44. A real swinger
_____ 45. Hump; humping	45. Spending $100
_____ 46. I got dinged	46. Doing jail or prison time
_____ 47. Ice it	47. Eat
_____ 48. I'm hip	48. Drunk

COLUMN A	COLUMN B
_____ 49. Joint	49. Innocent
_____ 50. Joneses	50. Not too smart; dumb
_____ 51. Jug	51. Sweet-talk a woman
_____ 52. Knocked	52. Money
_____ 53. Lame	53. Not too smart; dumb
_____ 54. Let's make it	54. Look over very well
_____ 55. Lid	55. The best
_____ 56. Man (the)	56. Stop
_____ 57. Mellow	57. Cadillac
_____ 58. Nailer	58. Stop
_____ 59. Not wired too heavy	59. Getting drunk; drinking
_____ 60. Not wrapped too tight	60. Not too smart; dumb
_____ 61. Oiled	61. Shut the window
_____ 62. Okey-dokey	62. Buy; get; steal
_____ 63. On the humble	63. Explain; squeal
_____ 64. Outa sight	64. Demoralized
_____ 65. Pad	65. Drunk
_____ 66. Peck	66. Shoes
_____ 67. Peek your hole card	67. Make an appearance
_____ 68. Piece	68. Doing something wrong
_____ 69. Popped	69. All right
_____ 70. Pressed	70. Slip around
_____ 71. Pull	71. Working the job
_____ 72. Pull a creep	72. Backed into a corner; tense
_____ 73. Put the check on	73. Lied; didn't keep his or her word
_____ 74. Put the hurt on you	74. Sweet talk failed
_____ 75. Rap; rapping	75. Hat
_____ 76. Regular	76. Dressed up
_____ 77. Ride	77. High
_____ 78. Run it down	78. Chair
_____ 79. Run it, man	79. Leave; go
_____ 80. Run you through a thing	80. Marijuana cigarette
_____ 81. Running game	81. Leave; go
_____ 82. Screaming	82. Especially good-looking woman

COLUMN A	COLUMN B
____ 83. Shank	83. Straighten up
____ 84. Shot a blank	84. Look over carefully
____ 85. Show	85. Policeman; white man in authority
____ 86. Smoothed out	86. Girl friend
____ 87. Something else	87. Policeman
____ 88. Split	88. Do you violence
____ 89. Steal you	89. Explain it
____ 90. Stomps	90. Trick you
____ 91. Stone fox	91. Conversation; talking
____ 92. Stone trick	92. Knife
____ 93. Stump	93. Car
____ 94. Take the cut	94. Talking
____ 95. Tap dancer	95. Tell it truthfully
____ 96. Tighten up	96. Leave; go
____ 97. Tore down	97. Sneak up behind you
____ 98. Tore up	98. Puzzling (can't figure out)
____ 99. Uptight	99. Didn't do right
____100. Wasted	100. Uncle Tom

EXPLANATION OF SCORING

Give yourself one point for each correct answer, and grade yourself according to the following scale:

100-90 = A

89-80 = B

79-70 = C

69-60 = D

Below 60 = F

ANSWERS

COLUMN A		COLUMN B		COLUMN A		COLUMN B
1	=	4		33	=	42
2	=	29		34	=	9
3	=	11		35	=	28
4	=	22, 92		36	=	20
5	=	40		37	=	59
6	=	39, 48, 65		38	=	33
7	=	31		39	=	7, 47
8	=	55		40	=	41, 93
9	=	10, 12, 52		41	=	19
10	=	38		42	=	27
11	=	54, 84		43	=	51
12	=	23		44	=	57
13	=	5		45	=	71
14	=	61		46	=	2
15	=	13		47	=	56, 58
16	=	44		48	=	26
17	=	62		49	=	80
18	=	1		50	=	43
19	=	63		51	=	37
20	=	14		52	=	18
21	=	30		53	=	36
22	=	6		54	=	35
23	=	15		55	=	75
24	=	45		56	=	85
25	=	46		57	=	86
26	=	10, 12, 52		58	=	87
27	=	34		59	=	50, 53, 60
28	=	10, 12, 52		60	=	50, 53, 60
29	=	50, 53, 60		61	=	39, 48, 65
30	=	25		62	=	3
31	=	21		63	=	49
32	=	56, 58		64	=	17

COLUMN A		COLUMN B		COLUMN A		COLUMN B
65	=	32		83	=	22, 92
66	=	7, 47		84	=	74
67	=	8		85	=	67
68	=	24		86	=	99
69	=	16		87	=	98
70	=	76		88	=	79, 81, 96
71	=	79, 81, 96		89	=	97
72	=	70		90	=	66
73	=	54, 84		91	=	82
74	=	88		92	=	73
75	=	91, 94		93	=	78
76	=	69		94	=	79, 81, 96
77	=	41, 93		95	=	100
78	=	95		96	=	83
79	=	89		97	=	39, 48, 65
80	=	90		98	=	77
81	=	68		99	=	72
82	=	91, 94		100	=	64

DISCUSSION GUIDELINES

1. What does your score indicate about your ability to understand numerous words and phrases that are commonly used by blacks?

2. Discuss this statement: "That a language system is different does not mean it is deficient."

3. What words and expressions in your vocabulary have been created by other groups in our culture? What do they mean?

4. In your family or group of friends do you have words or expressions that have private meanings (meanings for the family or friends only)? Where did they come from? What do they mean? What might be their effect on communication between the members of your family (or your friends) and members of another family (or another friendship group)?

Using Confrontation Effectively

A *confrontation* is a deliberate attempt to help another person to examine the consequences of some aspect of his or her behavior by sharing your perceptions of that behavior, its impact on you, and the inferences you draw about its motives and meaning. In an *informational* confrontation, you describe the visible behavior of another person. In an *interpretive* confrontation, you express what you think or feel about the meaning of another's behavior.

Six skills are involved in constructive confrontations:

1. The use of personal statements, *I, me, my,*

2. The use of relationship statements in which you express what you think or feel about the person with whom you are interacting,

3. The use of statements describing the visible behavior of the other person,

4. The use of descriptions of personal feelings specifying the feeling by name,

5. The use of understanding responses, such as paraphrasing and perception checking,

6. The use of constructive feedback skills.

The following learning activities offer you opportunities to practice confronting another person constructively. In each confrontation you should consciously apply the six confrontation skills. This activity is composed of three exercises that may be used separately or sequentially. Engaging in all three within a short period of time, however, may be an uncomfortably intense experience.

ROLE-PLAYING CONFRONTATIONS

Directions

1. Divide into triads. Designate one person as the confronter, another as the person being confronted, and the third as the observer.

Source: Reprinted from: Jones, John E., & Pfeiffer, J. William (Eds.). *The 1973 Annual Handbook for Group Facilitators.* La Jolla, CA: University Associates, 1973. Used with permission.

2. The group leader will assign a role-playing situation to each triad. The person being confronted plays the person described in the situation. The confronter tries to confront the other with as much authenticity and involvement as possible. The observer evaluates the effectiveness of the use of constructive confrontation, applying the six confrontation skills, as criteria.

3. After the confrontation has ended, the other two members of the triad give the confronter feedback on her or his use of the skills involved in constructive confrontation.

4. All three members switch roles and repeat the process with a different situation.

5. Again switch roles and repeat with a third situation.

Roles

The person being confronted plays the following role:

1. A person who is so "nice" that she or he is "unreal."

2. A person who constantly expresses a great deal of affection for everyone.

3. A person who jokes about other people's problems.

4. A person who frequently embarrasses others by making gross remarks and displaying bad table manners.

5. A person who is extremely shy in groups.

6. A person who often criticizes the behavior of others.

Discussion Guidelines

In the group as a whole, consider the following questions:

1. What did you learn about how you may confront other individuals more effectively?

2. What were your reactions to the exercise?

RELATIONSHIP CONFRONTATIONS

This exercise gives you an opportunity to use confrontation to improve the quality of your relationships.

Directions

1. Select a person with whom you have a good relationship. Between you, discuss the following issues, using the skills involved in constructive confrontation:

   a. "The things you do that most block our relationship are . . ."

   b. "The things you could do to improve our relationship are . . ."

2. At the end of fifteen minutes stop. Then choose another person with whom you have a good relationship. Again discuss these two issues.

3. At the end of fifteen minutes stop. Repeat the exercise with a third partner with whom you have a good relationship.

Discussion Guidelines

In the group as a whole, discuss your reactions to the exercise.

GOING AROUND THE CIRCLE

This exercise provides an opportunity for you to practice good confrontation skills with everyone in the group.

Directions

1. If you wish to participate in the exercise, form a circle with the other participants.

2. One at a time, you walk around the circle, stopping in front of each person. Look directly at the person, touch the person, and tell the person how you feel about her or him and your relationship.

Discussion Guidelines

After every participant has gone around the circle, discuss the following questions as a group:

1. What were your reactions to the exercise?

2. What did you learn about yourself and the other participants from it?

3. What could you do to improve your relationships with the other members of the group?

After completing all three exercises, you may wish to do a self-assessment in terms of confrontation skills. Check the appropriate statement:

_____ I have mastered constructively confronting other individuals.

_____ I need more work on constructively confronting other individuals.

39

Community Simulation

In a rural community of 50,000, the board of supervisors has scheduled a public meeting to determine how to allocate $3 million available to it from revenue sharing to meet the community's mental health needs. Members of the community (consumers and providers) have been invited to make presentations to the board identifying their needs and arguing their case for funding to meet these specific needs.

DIRECTIONS

1. Select a role you wish to play during the simulation (consumer, provider, or board member). There should be only three board members.

2. Meet with the others who have selected your role, and divide into groups each advocating a specific use of the funds.

3. With the other members of your group, prepare a presentation to make to the board. Include the following:

    a. A statement of the problems or needs.

    b. Identification of the target area and population (demographic data).

    c. Data to support your assertion of the existence and importance of the problems (statistical information, consumer demand, etc., including sources).

    d. Your request for funding.

    e. Your plan for use of the funds—the proposed program and evaluation method.

    The rationale for your proposal should reflect the principles of mental health planning.

4. Submit the presentation in writing to the board of supervisors.

5. Choose a speaker to represent the group in making an oral presentation to the board.

6. If you are chosen as speaker, make a presentation for no more than ten minutes.

Source: Adapted from materials developed by the faculty for students in community health nursing course, Department of Nursing, Sonoma State College, Rohnert Park, Calif., 1977.

7. If you are a member of the board of supervisors, evaluate the written and oral presentations of the groups with your fellow board members, and reach a decision about distributing the funds. Announce your decision, and explain the rationale for it.

DISCUSSION GUIDELINES

In the group as a whole, analyze the dynamics of the simulated experience, considering the following questions:

1. What were your reactions to the board's decision?

2. Which presentations were most influential with the board of supervisors? Why?

3. Which principles of mental health planning were applied in the simulation?

Drug Hazard Potentials:
An Exercise in Decision Making
by Consensus

Dr. Samuel Irwin, professor of psychopharmacology at the Medical School at the University of Oregon, has ranked twelve common drugs by their relative hazard potentials (overall potential for repeated or compulsive use, intravenous administration, self-destructive use, producing physical dependence and/or impaired judgment, predisposing to social deterioration, producing irreversible tissue damage and disease, and causing accidental death from overdose).* This exercise asks you to arrive at a similar ranking.

DIRECTIONS

In the chart below, individually rank the twelve drugs, placing the number 1 in column 1 beside the drug you believe is potentially most hazardous, 2 by your second choice, and so on. In a few instances, two drugs may tie for the same ranking.

Source: David W. Johnson and Frank P. Johnson, JOINING TOGETHER: Group Theory and Group Skills, ©1975, pp. 73-74, 323-25. Adapted by permission of Prentice-Hall, Inc., Englewood Cliffs, New Jersey.

*Samuel Irwin, "Drugs of Abuse: An Introduction to Their Actions and Potential Hazards," in *Starting Point*, a booklet published by the Florida State Department of Health and Rehabilitative Services.

DRUG	1 INDIVIDUAL RANKING	2 GROUP RANKING	3 EXPERT'S RANKING	DIFFERENCE BETWEEN 1 AND 3	DIFFERENCE BETWEEN 2 AND 3
Alcohol					
Barbiturates					
Tobacco (cigarette smoking)					
Dexedrine					
Glue sniffing					
Codeine					
Heroin					
Hypnotics					
LSD-25					
Marijuana					
Mescaline					
Methamphetamine					
			Total difference		

Divide into groups of about five and read the guidelines for consensus decisions.

Guidelines for Consensus Decisions

While consensus is the most effective method of group decision making, because of its high quality, it also takes the most time. Perfect consensus (with everyone in agreement about everything) is probably impossible to reach. However, other degrees of consensus can still bring about decisions of high quality. We can define *consensus* as a collective opinion, based on open and honest discussion among the members of a group, which the members publicly support (for at least a trial period). The following steps are important when striving for consensus:

1. Encourage *all* members of the group to participate.

2. Present your position as clearly and logically as possible.

3. Listen carefully to other members' positions and reactions, and consider them carefully.

4. Identify and consider the assumptions underlying your own position and that of others.

5. Yield to positions that are objective and logical.

6. Support suggestions or solutions with which you are in at least partial agreement.

7. Beware of changing your mind simply because you want to reduce conflict or disagreement.

8. Encourage the expression of differences of opinion. Such differences give the group more information, increasing its chances to make effective decisions.

9. Avoid using conflict-reducing techniques such as majority vote, tossing a coin, finding an average, or bargaining.

10. Avoid stalemates by looking for the next most acceptable alternative.

Following these guidelines, rank the drugs, working as a group, using the consensus method of decision making. You have thirty minutes to reach a set of group consensus scores. Enter these scores in column 2 on the chart.

EXPLANATION OF SCORING

The ranking according to Dr. Irwin is:

___3___ Alcohol   ___6___ Heroin

___5___ Barbiturates   ___5___ Hypnotics

___4___ Tobacco (cigarette smoking)   ___7___ LSD-25

___2___ Dexedrine   ___8___ Marijuana

___1___ Glue sniffing   ___7___ Mescaline

___6___ Codeine   ___2___ Methamphetamine

Enter these scores in column 3 on the chart and complete the last two columns. Compare your individual total difference with that of the group.

Experts Rationale

Glue sniffing was rated highest because it leads to rapid loss of control and consciousness, possible overdosage, and death from respiratory arrest. It can also produce irreversible damage to the brain and bodily tissues.

Methamphetamine and dexedrine (or "speed"), especially when taken intravenously were rated second because of their high psychological dependence risk (they are too pleasurable). They also predictably produce a paranoid schizophrenic state with greatly impaired judgment, excitement, and a tendency for violence after repeated use of doses three or more times what a physician might prescribe. Taking the drug by injection leads to further impairment of functioning, a possibility of hepatitis and of septicemia from the use of unsterile materials, and a probable need for protective hospitalization.

Alcohol was ranked third because it has high potentials for psychological dependence, greatly impairs judgment and coordination (a leading cause of driving accidents), increases aggressiveness and violent behavior, often produces marked social deterioration, and causes irreversible damage to the brain, liver, and other body issues. The withdrawal symptoms (delirium tremens) from alcohol abuse are also often life-threatening and difficult to treat.

Tobacco (cigarette smoking) is listed next (fourth) because of the high incidence of irreversible damage (to lungs, heart, and blood vessels) and cancer formation accompanying its prolonged use. These hazards greatly reduce the life span and often debilitate the individual long before death.

Barbiturates and hypnotics were ranked fifth because, although similar to alcohol in their overall effects and dependence liabilities, they do not cause as much extensive tissue damage. A greater danger with the hypnotics, however, is the increased possibility of death from overdose.

Heroin was rated sixth because, unlike alcohol and barbiturates, it does not impair coordination and judgment in normal doses, does not produce extensive tissue damage, and is more likely to inhibit aggressive behavior. When taken intravenously, it is potentially very addictive, both psychologically and physically, and continued use can lead to social deterioration. But the physical dependence would be of relatively little consequence if the drug were available. Sufficient tolerance develops to the depressant effects so that it is possible to function more productively under the influence of heroin than with alcohol or barbiturates. The main danger from heroin (or morphine) is acute respiratory failure and death from overdose among inexperienced users, as a very narrow margin exists between the effective dose and the lethal dose. With illicit supplies varying greatly in potency, this is a serious danger. Because unsterile materials are often used for injection, there is also a risk of hepatitis and septicemia.

LSD-25 is seventh on the list because, although it can cause psychotic reactions, such occurrences are relatively rare (less than 1 percent of volunteers in clinical settings have prolonged adverse reactions; and the rate of psychotic reactions for the general population of illicit users is probably less than 5 percent). LSD is not addictive in the usual sense; it is taken intermittently and usually gradually discontinued. The hallucinogens produce no physical dependence but pose hazards in individuals, and flashbacks of effects may occur even months after the last dose (attributed by some physicians to hysterical reactions associated with unresolved conflicts). The lethal dose is so high that no human deaths have been reported from overdosage.

Marijuana is ranked last in intrinsic hazard because there have been fewer untoward reactions from its use requiring hospitalization than from any other psychoactive drug. Marijuana is more apt to reduce aggressiveness than to increase it. Psychological dependence is not as great a hazard as with alcohol; there is little tolerance development, no danger of physiological dependence, and no significant tissue damage. In small and moderate doses there seems to be only minor impairment of judgment or coordination. The lethal dose is so high that it is extremely difficult to kill oneself from overdose.

DISCUSSION GUIDELINES

On a chalkboard, list the difference scores for each group. Have members of the group who achieved the lowest difference score describe how the group functioned in reaching consensus. Discuss how the functioning of other, less effective groups differed. Consider the following questions:

1. What was the interpersonal climate within the group?

2. Did members feel listened to?

3. Were they able to influence the decisions?

4. How committed to the group decision do members feel?

Guide to Interaction Process Analysis

In order to learn the function of therapeutic intervention, the process of a therapeutic nurse-client relationship, you must be able to study and review with objectivity the components of this process. As the responsible individual in the interaction, you must review both verbal and nonverbal components for their potential meaning. They may be expressing problems or attempts at resolving problems. The tool used for this review is the *interaction process analysis*. An IPA is a verbatim and progressive recording of the verbal and nonverbal interactions between client and nurse within a given period of time. It consists of:

1. A summary of the circumstances associated with the recorded interaction.

2. An accurate and objective recording of the verbal and behavioral communication between client and nurse within the period. It may describe nonverbal communication alone, if conversation does not occur. If conversation does occur, the IPA must both record the words and describe accompanying nonverbal communication by each participant in the interaction. Nonverbal behavior is described in parentheses. Exchanges must be recorded in proper sequence, to indicate the direction of the communication.

3. For each significant communication (verbal or nonverbal), a statement in the nurse- or the client-centered analysis (or both) that specifies the following:

   a. An analysis or interpretation of the possible meaning of the communication,

   b. Identification of the nurse's own emotions and the possible intent of the nurse's communication, whether conscious or unconscious,

   c. Perceptions of the emotions expressed by the client and the intent of the client's communication, whether conscious or unconscious,

   d. Evaluation of the effectiveness of the nurse's approach, based on the above data,

   e. Suggestions of nursing alternatives in order of their usefulness.

DIRECTIONS

Prepare an interaction process analysis for each of several sessions with your client. Before filling out the form the first time, duplicate sufficient copies of it for each use.

INTERACTION PROCESS ANALYSIS

Circumstances

Description of environmental setting:

Feeling tone
   Nurse's:

   Client's:

Unit milieu:

Description of client:

Significant data prior to interaction:

Goals
   Nurse-centered:

Client-centered:

Interaction Process Analysis

INTERACTION *(Verbal and Nonverbal)*	*NURSE-CENTERED ANALYSIS*	*CLIENT-CENTERED ANALYSIS*

INTERACTION (VERBAL AND NONVERBAL)	NURSE-CENTERED ANALYSIS	CLIENT-CENTERED ANALYSIS

Summary

Themes perceived in interaction:

Evaluation in terms of goals
  Nurse-centered goals:

Client-centered goals:

References to theory (articles or books read as preparation for IPA):

Seating Arrangements in Groups

DIRECTIONS

1. Complete this tool for each session of a group therapy series. Before filling out the form the first time, duplicate sufficient copies of it for each use.

2. In the space above the chart, draw a seating diagram, viewed from above the room. Draw the walls of the room and show the arrangement of the furniture (sofas, easy chairs, straight chairs, desks, tables, etc.). Show the positions of doors and windows.

3. Identify each chair with the name of the group member occupying it.

4. Designate empty chairs with an X.

5. Use arrows to indicate how any group member alters his or her seating position during a session.

6. Use the chart to record whether members are present, absent, or late and to keep a cumulative total of absences and latenesses by each member.

7. For every group session, answer the questions that follow the chart.

SEATING DIAGRAM

Session number:

Date:

147

NAME OF GROUP MEMBER	PRESENT OR ABSENT	TOTAL NUMBER OF TIMES ABSENT	ON TIME OR LATE	NUMBER OF MINUTES LATE	TOTAL NUMBER OF TIMES LATE

QUESTIONS

1. What leadership activities have you undertaken about absences in specific instances? What was your rationale? What was the outcome?

2. What leadership activities have you undertaken about tardiness in specific instances? What was your rationale? What was the outcome?

3. What sense can you make of members' choices of seating?

4. How does the physical setting, including seating, influence group interaction?

Understanding Silence

This tool may be used to help you understand silence in therapeutic encounters.

DIRECTIONS

In the form below, note your observations about the quality and quantity of the silence that occurs in sessions with a client and the verbal and nonverbal behavior of both client and therapist. Analyze the silences according to the guidelines that follow the form.

Complete this tool a total of five times, after reviewing your data from:

1. The first session with the client (whether individual, group, or family).

2. The second session.

3. The final session.

4. Any other two sessions.

Before filling out the form the first time, duplicate sufficient copies of it for each use.

LENGTH AND FEELING TONE OF SILENCE	VERBAL AND NONVERBAL DATA PRECEDING, DURING, AND AFTER SILENCE	THERAPIST RESPONSES (THOUGHTS, FEELINGS, ACTIONS)

ANALYSIS GUIDELINES

In the space below, analyze the silences by comparing therapeutic sessions. Is there a trend in terms of the client's responses? What is it? What is the significance of silence with this client? Is there a pattern to your responses? What is it? What is the significance of your pattern of responses to the client?

Sociodrama Participant's Guide

A *sociodrama* is an action-oriented laboratory exercise for observing verbal and nonverbal communication and for studying and solving problems in interpersonal relationships. It focuses on the interactions between people. You can use it:

1. To learn why a nursing approach or action was ineffective.

2. To explore and try out alternative approaches.

3. To become more creative in working with clients.

4. To increase your understanding of your interpersonal dynamics.

DIRECTIONS

As a class, conduct a sociodrama session. Begin by suggesting sociodrama problems. Each problem should be:

1. One in which you were actually involved.

2. One in which you are dissatisfied with your approach or behavior.

3. One you want to explore further in order to find a more satisfactory solution.

4. One related to a specific situation with specific time limits.

Suggestions may include nurse-client problems, problems with coworkers (nursing, medical, and other personnel), problems with relatives of patients, etc.

The content of the session must be held strictly confidential. What takes place cannot be discussed outside. You are thus free to use the actual names of those who are characters in your sociodrama problem.

The instructor will help to organize and terminate the drama and lead the discussion.

1. As a group, select one of the problems suggested to focus on.

2. If you are the person whose situation was selected, request volunteer actors from the group to portray the significant persons in the situation.

3. Brief the actors on their roles, outside the room.

4. Return to the room, and describe the setting to the audience. Indicate what role each actor is playing. You will play yourself in the sociodrama.

5. With the other actors, reenact the situation. You may use props. Attempt to capture the mood and tone of the characters and scene rather than to reproduce the exact dialogue, ad lib while trying to maintain the mood.

6. If you are not the person whose problem is selected, and you are not chosen as an actor, you are a member of the audience. Record the proceedings (see activity 45, next). During the enactment, observe both verbal and nonverbal behaviors of the participants.

7. When the drama is terminated, relate what you saw and heard going on in the interchange, and indicate the feeling tones you detected in the nurse and the actors. You may also indicate your observations on how the relationship opened, the turning point, the "controlling" person, what the nurse's goal was and whether it was accomplished, and how the relationship ended.

8. If you were one of the actors, describe your feelings during the presentation of the problem.

9. Anyone may then suggest a different nursing approach and may volunteer to portray it. If your problem was enacted, you yourself may portray the alternative. You may continue to portray the same alternative until you become comfortable with it. Actors may reverse their roles (nurse playing client and vice versa, for example) or new cast members may be selected according to suggestions from the participants, the audience, or the instructor.

Sociodrama Observer's Guide

DIRECTIONS

Complete the form below as an observer in a sociodrama session (see activity 44).

Date: Session number:

Notes on Selection

Problems suggested (brief summary):

Selected Problem:

Student presenting problem:

Volunteer actor or actors:

Notes on Enactment

Verbal behavior:

Nonverbal behavior:

Feeling tones:

Opening of relationship:

Controlling person:

Turning point:

Subject's goals and extent of accomplishment:

Other significant observations:

Closing of relationship:

Notes on Discussion

Issues during discussion (specify initiator of issue):

Nursing alternatives offered:

Nursing alternative selected:

Comments:

Literature as a Means to Understanding: Total Institutions

This activity stimulates you to explore the characteristics of total institutions and the processes of institutionalization by critically analyzing fiction and nonfiction works on these subjects.

DIRECTIONS

Read the following:

1. Erving Goffman, *Asylums* (Garden City, N.Y.: Doubleday Anchor Books, 1961), pp. xiii, 1-124.

2. Ken Kesey, *One Flew Over the Cuckoo's Nest* (New York: New American Library, Signet Edition, 1966).

DISCUSSION GUIDELINES

Engage in a small group discussion of the following questions:

1. In the total institution as discussed by Goffman, enforced activities are brought together into a single rational plan purportedly designed to fulfill the official aim of the institution. What do you think the ultimate aim of Kesey's "Big Nurse" is, based on what you observe about the enforced activities on her ward?

2. In total institutions, Goffman asserts, there is a basic split between a large managed group called *inmates* and a small supervisory staff. What in Kesey's novel might symbolize this split or distance?

3. A characteristic of total institutions is a demoralized work system. Can you cite an example of such a system from Kesey's novel?

4. In our society, total institutions, according to Goffman's framework, are the forcing houses for changing persons: each institution is an experiment about what can be done with the self. This idea is discussed to a great extent by Bromden in *Cuckoo's Nest*.

What is Bromden's name for the concept? Can you cite some evidence to support it from Kesey's novel?

5. Upon entering a total institution, inmates are immediately stripped of their "presenting culture." This is the first in a series of abasements, degradations, and humiliations of the self they undergo. What about McMurphy's admission process captures this attempt on the part of the total institution?

6. Both Goffman and Kesey discuss admission procedures. "The new arrival allows himself to be coded into an object that can be fed into the administrative machinery of the establishment," says Goffman. What are some examples of admission procedures from *Cuckoo's Nest?*

7. Mortification, according to Goffman, occurs when inmates expose their interpersonal relationships and when they take no action when an assault is made upon a fellow inmate. An example quoted in *Asylums* is Herman Melville's description of flogging in the British navy (p. 34). Goffman comments that "all conveys a terrible hint of the omnipotent authority under which [the inmate] lives." Give a clear example of mortification in this form from *Cuckoo's Nest.*

8. Regimentation and tyranny are characteristic of total institutions. Autonomy of action is violated, and inmates are not permitted to schedule their own activities. Cite examples of this from Big Nurse's ward.

9. Goffman notes that inmates may be considered so insignificant in status by staff that they are not given even minor greetings. How does Bromden's "deafness" relate to this observation?

10. The "privilege system" of the total institution represents the framework for the inmate's personal reorganization after stripping occurs. Punishments in this system are the consequences of breaking the rules. How might McMurphy's brief withdrawal from "the battle" be considered in this context?

11. Can you think of examples in Kesey's novel of "messing up" as defined by Goffman? What were the consequences for those involved?

12. Institutional ceremonies that occur through such media as the house organ, group meetings, open house programs, and charitable performances presumably fulfill latent social functions, according to Goffman. However, he goes on to state that often there is a hint of rebellion in the role the inmates take. They use these ceremonies as opportunities in which subordinates can in some way profane superordinates. When and how does this occur in Kesey's novel?

13. Goffman comments that the contradiction between what the institution does and what its officials say it does forms the basic context of the staff's daily activity. Do you see this contradiction in *Cuckoo's Nest* when the public relations man visits the ward? How is it illustrated by what goes on in the "therapeutic group meetings"?

14. The obligation of the staff to maintain certain humane standards of treatment for inmates presents problems in itself, but a further set of characteristic problems is found in the constant conflict between humane standards and organizational efficiency. Just as personal possessions may interfere with smooth running of an institutional operation and be removed for this reason, so parts of the body may also conflict with efficient management, and the conflict may be resolved in favor of efficiency. This occurs in

Kesey's novel on a symbolic level with Billy Bibbit and more explicitly in the case of McMurphy. What happens?

15. Often the privileges and punishments that the staff mete out are phrased in language that reflects the legitimated objectives of the institution. This practice is basic to the means of social control. In these terms, how does McMurphy threaten the control of Big Nurse?

47

Simulated Family Experience

This role-playing interaction is designed to help you

1. Recognize the organization, energy use, and role patterns in a family system,

2. Identify communication and adaptation patterns in the family system, and

3. Explore the value of analyzing a family from a systems theory perspective.

DIRECTIONS

1. Five family roles and an event are presented below. The class leader will select individuals to play each role.

2. If you are chosen for a role, enact the scene set by the family event with the other family members. Take ten minutes for the simulation.

3. If you are not playing a role, observe the simulation and consider the questions for discussion.

Roles

Mother in midthirties

Father in midthirties

Sixteen-year-old daughter

Fourteen-year-old daughter

Twelve-year-old daughter

Source: Developed by the faculty for students in community health nursing course, Department of Nursing, Sonoma State College, Rohnert Park, Calif., 1977.

Family Event

The oldest daughter took the family car, with her parents' permission, and arrived home late. She took her two sisters with her without her parents' knowledge.

DISCUSSION GUIDELINES

As a class, consider the following aspects of the simulation:

1. How was energy used in the family?

2. What types of roles emerged? Who assumed what roles?

3. Was there any evidence of role conflict? What was it?

4. Who made decisions in the family? Who assumed leadership?

48

Feedback Rating Exercise

Feedback from others is the primary means by which you can increase your self-awareness. Since your ability to self-disclose depends on your self-awareness, it is important for you to receive as much feedback as possible. You need to have others tell you their impressions of you and how they are reacting to your behavior in the group. They can do this simply by stating, "My impression of you is . . . ," or "My reactions to your behavior are . . . ," or "The way I feel about you is . . . ."

Sometimes you may be unsure what your impressions are of another person or how you are reacting to someone's behavior. One way to clarify your impressions and reactions is to associate some animal, bird, song, color, type of weather, movie, book, food, or fantasy with the person. You may ask yourself, "What animal do I associate with this person: a puppy, a fox, a bear?" "What books do I associate with this person?" Or "what songs do I associate with this person?" Finally, you may wish to ask, "What fantasies do I associate with this man? Do I see him as a knight in shining armor, an innkeeper in medieval England, a French chef, a conforming business executive, a professional singer?" By telling someone what animal, song, color, etc., you associate with him or her, you may clarify your impressions and reactions and provide the other person with interesting, entertaining, and helpful feedback.

The scale in this exercise is designed to help you learn more about your feedback style.

DIRECTIONS

The scales below list the opposite extremes on several dimensions of the style of giving feedback. For each item, draw a circle around the number that best characterizes where your feedback style lies between the extremes.

Sources: Reprinted from: Pfeiffer, J. William, & Jones, John E. (Eds.), *A Handbook of Structured Experiences for Human Relations Training*, Volume III. La Jolla, CA: University Associates, 1971. Used with permission. David W. Johnson, REACHING OUT: Interpersonal Effectiveness and Self-Actualization, ©1972, p. 33. Adapted by permission of Prentice-Hall, Inc., Englewood Cliffs, New Jersey.

Indirect Expression of Feeling Not describing your own emotional state, e.g., "You are a very likable person."	1 2 3 4 5	*Direct Expression of Feeling* Describing your own emotional state, e.g., "I like you very much."
Attributive Feedback Ascribing motives to the other person's behavior, e.g., "You are angry with me."	1 2 3 4 5	*Descriptive Feedback* Observing and describing the behavior to which you are reacting, e.g., "You are frowning, and your hands are clenched in a fist."
Evaluative Feedback Passing judgment on another person's behavior or imposing your standards, e.g., "You shouldn't be so angry."	1 2 3 4 5	*Nonevaluative Feedback* Commenting on behavior without judging its worth or value, e.g., "It seems to me you're very angry about that."
General Feedback Stating broad reactions and not indicating specific behaviors, e.g., "You're pretty touchy today."	1 2 3 4 5	*Specific Feedback* Pointing out the specific actions to which you are reacting, e.g., "When you frowned, I felt anxious."
Pressure on the Other to Change Implying that people are not behaving according to your standards, e.g., "Don't call me 'kid'—it's patronizing."	1 2 3 4 5	*Expression of Own Negative Reactions* Describing your negative feelings and allowing others to decide whether they want to change their behavior, e.g., "When you called me 'kid,' I felt put down."
Delayed Feedback Postponing feedback on others' behavior until later, e.g., "I was really hurt yesterday when you ignored me."	1 2 3 4 5	*Immediate Feedback* Responding immediately after the event, e.g., "I'm feeling hurt because you're not responding to me."
External Feedback Focusing attention on events outside the group, e.g., "My friends see me as being very supportive."	1 2 3 4 5	*Group-shared Feedback* Focusing attention on events that occur in the group, e.g., "Do the members of this group see me as being very supportive?"

DISCUSSION GUIDELINES

Divide into groups of four or five and share your ratings.

1. How would the members of your group rate your feedback style?

2. Giving feedback effectively is a skill that can be developed. On the basis of your own ratings and the feedback from other group members, which items do you want to work on further? Ask for continuing feedback from the group on those items.

49

Clinical Diaries: An In-Depth Analysis of Small Group Processes

A clinical diary can be used as a tool for analyzing what is going on in a small therapy group, identifying problems, and evaluating your leadership approaches as therapist. The diary is not a log of all interactions that take place during a session, but rather a narrative *summary* of the session's events, in clear, concise, chronological terms, focused on a particular topic. In the diary, you also apply psychiatric theory to the description of the group session and analyze the group conceptually in terms of the topic selected.

DIRECTIONS

Keep a clinical diary for a series of group therapy sessions in which you are serving as leader or cotherapist. Choose as a topic or focus for the diary a problem you want to explore in depth about your group. Topics often chosen include:

1. The cotherapist contract. What rules have you and your coleader agreed on? What impact do they have on the group?

2. The group contract. How did the group arrive at its ground rules? What are some of them? How well are they working?

3. Starting and/or closing the group. What are the important considerations at these points in the group's life? How are you handling them?

4. Group leading techniques. What approaches characterize your intervention and participation in the group? Are they effective? If not, why not?

5. Group processes. What are the dominant processes in the group (e.g., resistance, cohesion, conflict, inclusion, monopolizing, silence, termination, here-and-now interactions). What conclusions can you draw about the group process and dynamics?

6. Group organization. How are you handling the establishment of the group in terms of considerations such as size, membership, seating arrangements, and the like?

Source: Adapted from materials developed by the faculty for students in interaction and change nursing course, Department of Nursing, Sonoma State College, Rohnert Park, Calif., 1977.

In the diary for each session, include the following sections:

1. A narrative description of the session, focusing on the topic. Relate what happened in terms of the subject you are exploring.

2. A review of the literature on the topic. Refer to at least three authorities that illuminate the topic, and explain their ideas.

3. An analysis of the topic and the experts' ideas about it. Break the subject down for close examination. Weigh the authorities' opinions for appropriateness, situational characteristics, biases, mistakes, strengths, etc.

4. A conclusion. Based on the preceding sections and your own thinking, put together a new picture of your group in terms of the topic you chose as a focus. Include creative thinking, new insights, plans for the next session, and your assessment of what you did well.

Submit your diary to your instructor or clinical supervisor for evaluation and discussion.

Group Coleaders' Inventory

This tool is designed to help you establish and maintain an egalitarian coleading relationship.

DIRECTIONS

Before beginning a group therapy experience with a coleader, complete tasks 1 through 5. Your coleader should do the same.

1. In the space below, write approximately 100 words explaining your concept of how group therapy helps people. Refer to the theorists and theories that guide your work.

2. List at least ten things that you expect to happen in the group you will be coleading. Identify the very *worst*, and the very *best* things that could happen.

EXPECTATIONS	
BEST POSSIBILITY	*WORST POSSIBILITY*

3. Complete the following statements about your typical responses in therapeutic work with clients:

When beginning the relationship, I usually

When someone talks too much, I usually

When a client is silent, I usually

When someone cries, I usually

When someone comes late, I usually

When people are excessively polite and unwilling to confront each other, I usually

When there is conflict in a group, I usually

When one individual is verbally attacked, I usually

If there is physical violence, I usually

When clients discuss sexual feelings about others, or about me, I usually

My "favorite" interventions are

My typical intervention "rhythm" (fast/slow) is

My style is characteristically more (nurturing/confronting)

The thing that makes me most uncomfortable in groups is

4. Complete the information below on your past group experiences

APPROXIMATE DATES	DURATION	TYPE OF GROUP	MY ROLE

5. List your scores from self-assessment instruments, such as activities 1, 5, 6, 8, and 12 of this workbook, that have helped you understand yourself better. Comment on what these data mean in terms of an egalitarian coleader relationship.

Exchange the above responses with your coleader. Share your reactions to the exchange of information and elaborate for each other where necessary.

Together complete tasks 6 through 13.

6. Do activity 51, "Coleader Encounter," next in this workbook.

7. State some of your coleader behavior patterns, and indicate the behaviors your coleader might see as idiosyncratic.

8. Describe the personal growth efforts that you are making right now. Indicate what personal growth goals you anticipate working on during this group experience.

9. Note issues that have arisen in your past work with other coleaders.

10. Discuss your reactions to the makeup of the group, its size, and any other special considerations.

11. Set up operating norms and a coleader contract:

   a. Where will you each sit in the group meetings?

   b. Who will begin and end each session?

   c. How will lateness and absence be handled?

   d. How much "there-and-then" discussion will be allowed, and how do you define "here-and-now"?

   e. Will you make theory inputs? If so, how?

   f. What will you do about group members' requests for contacts outside the group?

12. Discuss your anticipated coleading style:

   a. Where, when, and how will you deal with issues between the two of you?

   b. Can you agree to disagree?

   c. Will you encourage or discourage conflict?

    d. How much of your behavior will be role-determined, and how much will be personal and individual?

    e. Is it possible for you to use each other's energy—that is, can one of you be "out" while the other is "in"?

    f. How will you establish and maintain growth-producing norms?

    g. What is nonnegotiable for each of you as coleader?

13. Discuss your ethics:

    a. What responsibilities do you each have after the group experience is over? Are you responsible for referral?

    b. What responsibilities do you have for screening?

    c. Are you adequately qualified? How have you communicated your qualifications to the group?

    d. What are your standards with regard to confidentiality?

After each group session, complete tasks 14 through 16.

14. Analyze the group:

    a. On a ten-point scale, how did things go in this meeting?

    b. What is happening in the group?

    c. Is anyone "hurting"?

    d. What are the themes?

    e. Which group dynamics are operative?

15. Solicit feedback from each other by asking:

    a. What did I do that was effective?

    b. What did I do that was ineffective?

    c. How am I working as a coleader?

    d. What else would you like from me that I'm not giving?

16. Consider renegotiating the coleadership contract:

    a. Is there anything that you need to renegotiate?

    b. How are you feeling about each other?

    c. What is each of you going to do in the next group meeting?

After the final group session, complete task 17.

17. Terminate the coleading relationship:

    a. Discuss the extent to which your personal goals were achieved.

    b. Discuss under what conditions you would work together again.

    c. Discuss your personal and professional learning from this experience.

d. Solicit ideas for your continued personal growth.

e. Solicit ideas about improving your group-leading competence.

Coleader Encounter

When you communicate with another person, your responses are formed by your perceptions of that person. In other words, when you talk to another, you are actually talking to an image you have of that person. Your image may not be the same as the image the person has of himself or herself.

In order to establish a mutual world with another, you need to find out about the "real" other person, to obtain an accurate picture of that person's self-image. What questions should you ask in order to obtain an accurate perception? This exercise is designed to help you find out.

DIRECTIONS

Below list ten questions your coleader should ask in order to know the "real" you. Exchange lists with your coleader. You have thirty minutes in which to interview each other using the questions your coleader has provided to achieve the most self-disclosure. Write out your coleader's answers to her or his ten questions. Your coleader will write down your answers to your questions. Discuss your answers with one another.

1.

2.

3.

4.

5.

6.

7.

8.

9.

10.

Analyzing a Crisis Call

DIRECTIONS

Analyze the following verbatim recording of a call taken by a nurse at a crisis intervention center. In making your analysis, refer to activity 41, "Guide to Interaction Process Analysis." The conversation is presented in the IPA format.

Interaction Process Analysis

INTERACTION (VERBAL AND NONVERBAL)	NURSE-CENTERED ANALYSIS	CLIENT-CENTERED ANALYSIS
Nurse: Can I help you?		
Caller: Yes, you may (crying).		
Nurse: You sound pretty upset. What seems to be the problem?		
Caller: I don't know. It's just too much to go on.		
Nurse: What's going on now that seems like too much?		
Caller: My mother just died.		
Nurse: Your mother just died?		
Caller: Yes.		
Nurse: When was that?		

INTERACTION (VERBAL AND NONVERBAL)	NURSE-CENTERED ANALYSIS	CLIENT-CENTERED ANALYSIS
Caller (crying): Excuse me. About a week ago.		
Nurse: Wow—that's pretty upsetting, isn't it?		
Caller: I just can't take any more bad things happening to me (crying).		
Nurse: What else has been happening to you?		
Caller: All kinds of problems.		
Nurse: Like what?		
Caller: Boys and parties and all sorts of stuff. (Cries.) I don't know what to do.		
Nurse: You're feeling really low now, aren't you?		
Caller: Pardon?		
Nurse: You're feeling really low now.		
Caller: Yes.		
Nurse: How do you feel about your mother's death?		
Caller: Alone. My father doesn't want me.		
Nurse: What?		
Caller: My father doesn't want me.		
Nurse: Where are you going to end up then?		

INTERACTION (VERBAL AND NONVERBAL)	NURSE-CENTERED ANALYSIS	CLIENT-CENTERED ANALYSIS
Caller: I don't know.		
Nurse: Your father doesn't want you?		
Caller: No.		
Nurse: How do you know?		
Caller: He said so.		
Nurse: Can you tell me your name?		
Caller: No.		
Nurse: Just your first name?		
Caller: No.		
Nurse: Okay. Who are you staying with now?		
Caller: My aunt.		
Nurse: So your aunt wants you.		
Caller: Yes—I guess so.		
Nurse: How long have you been staying with her?		
Caller: About a couple of days.		
Nurse: So you haven't stayed with your father in a few days, is that it?		
Caller: Yes.		
Nurse: That's . . . that's pretty . . . that's pretty damn upsetting.		

INTERACTION (VERBAL AND NONVERBAL)	NURSE-CENTERED ANALYSIS	CLIENT-CENTERED ANALYSIS
Caller: It is; it sure is.		
Nurse: To know that your father doesn't want you. I don't blame you for crying about that.		
Caller: What?		
Nurse: I said I don't blame you for crying about that.		
Caller: I just don't know what to do, I can't stand it.		
Nurse: How long have you been feeling like this?		
Caller: Oh, for a long time.		
Nurse: Do you have any other brothers and sisters?		
Caller: No.		
Nurse: You're the only child?		
Caller: Yes.		
Nurse: Do you know why he doesn't want you?		
Caller: No. (crying).		
Nurse: He didn't tell you?		
Caller: No. He just didn't give me any reason. He wants to go his own way (crying).		
Nurse: That's . . . that's hurt your feelings.		
Caller: Yes.		

INTERACTION (VERBAL AND NONVERBAL)	NURSE-CENTERED ANALYSIS	CLIENT-CENTERED ANALYSIS
Nurse: What is he doing now? Caller: I don't know. Nurse: You haven't heard from him? Caller: No. Nurse: In how long? Caller: In a very long time . . . . (Hangs up.)		

53

Analyzing an Individual Session

DIRECTIONS

Analyze the following verbatim recording of a second session with a client in individual relationship therapy. In making your analysis, refer to activity 41, "Guide to Interaction Process Analysis."

The client, Jennie, is a twenty-six-year-old woman who lives with her five-year-old daughter. Scott, her husband, moved out of the house last month. Jennie was briefly hospitalized in a psychiatric unit three years ago with a diagnosis of "obsessive-compulsive reaction."

Interaction Process Analysis

INTERACTION (VERBAL AND NONVERBAL)	NURSE-CENTERED ANALYSIS	CLIENT-CENTERED ANALYSIS
(Jennie arrives fifteen minutes late.) Nurse: Hi, Jennie. Jennie: Hi. The cab was a little late. Nurse: You took a cab? Jennie: Yeah. It's freezing out and I knew that . . . I . . . didn't feel like walking up (laugh), plus I . . . I was . . . um . . . (quietly) getting ready at the last minute, anyway.		

189

© 1979 by Addison-Wesley Publishing Company, Inc.

INTERACTION (VERBAL AND NONVERBAL)	NURSE-CENTERED ANALYSIS	CLIENT-CENTERED ANALYSIS
Nurse: Ah hum. Sometimes have trouble getting going?		
Jennie: Yes!		
(Silence.)		
Nurse: So how are things going?		
Jennie: Um . . . last night . . . not so well.		
Nurse: Not so well?		
Jennie: Oh . . . (low voice) I don't know, I guess. It happened after I ate dinner. I just, I don't know if it's the low blood sugar or nerves or what. I mean it *acts* like low blood sugar.		
Nurse: How's that? You mentioned this before—with low blood sugar you have certain symptoms, and you feel like you know when it's happening. How does it feel?		
Jennie: Well . . . like, first, I guess, first I notice that my thinking was getting worse. And, like, it was harder to *think* and harder to concentrate. And, like, I never realized . . . I thought some of that business was just emotions and being upset, and then, after reading this book I have on low blood sugar, it explains that . . . like, if your blood sugar is low, well it's low for your whole body, so		

INTERACTION (VERBAL AND NONVERBAL)	NURSE-CENTERED ANALYSIS	CLIENT-CENTERED ANALYSIS
your brain is only half nourished, like, with sugar— (quietly) so it's just not going to work as well. So . . . you know . . . it's probably that. But I guess emotions can trigger off stuff like that, too. But, then, food has something to do with it, cause they put you on a special diet, you know, and . . . but then . . . once your blood sugar gets low, you can get . . . like, I started to get real irritable and feeling depressed and . . . um . . . then my ears get real sensitive to noise—like the kids were playing . . . and they weren't that loud, I'm sure . . . ah . . . but it started pounding in my ears, and then I had to leave the room, it hurt so bad. Nurse: Um hum. Jennie: But all the symptoms were of low blood sugar. The doctor doesn't know what's causing it, you know . . . ah . . . I guess a lot of times they don't know, and then sometimes they can find out? Nurse: Yes, I would think the physical and emotional could both be contributing, and this may be an area we'll want to sort out more clearly—perhaps have some physical work done soon. I wonder if we could look at the emotional question for a time here, though . . . I'm wondering, Jennie, when did all these feelings start yesterday? What time of day was it?		

INTERACTION (VERBAL AND NONVERBAL)	NURSE-CENTERED ANALYSIS	CLIENT-CENTERED ANALYSIS
Jennie: Ah, it was after supper.		
Nurse: And before that time you were feeling—how?		
Jennie: Ah, I wasn't real good, I was . . . um . . . I wasn't all that irritable or anything, but I was having trouble concentrating and thinking, which I have most all the time.		
Nurse: Ah huh.		
Jennie: It's just like . . . (surprised) Well, the day before I was thinking good! I was thinking more clearly.		
Nurse: Were you anticipating something happening?		
Jennie: Well, Scott was supposed to call that night, that's the only thing I can think of that would make me a little nervous. But actually I didn't really want to see him 'cause I wasn't thinking that clearly. The night before I was thinking good and I thought I *could talk* to him. But then last night—yesterday—I wasn't thinking all that well . . . . I don't think I slept good the night before . . . um . . . but (quietly) I don't know exactly why I wasn't sleeping good, whether it was that, I don't know.		
Nurse: Jennie, I'm wondering— what feelings you were having last night. Was it a fearful feeling?		

INTERACTION (VERBAL AND NONVERBAL)	NURSE-CENTERED ANALYSIS	CLIENT-CENTERED ANALYSIS
Jennie: Um . . . (long pause). No. I had those . . . um, not really. I don't think it was. Maybe it was a little bit . . . um . . . well, maybe because of it I felt afraid that . . . er . . . because (slower, very quiet) I don't like to be sick like that.		
Nurse: Ah huh?		
Jennie: But I . . . I don't really know . . . . I wouldn't say it was really *fear*, but it . . . bothered me that I felt like that. But, but I have had fear at other times . . . like . . . going to sleep and . . . well, I don't know if it's fear or rejection or what—you know, but . . . thinking about Scott . . . (eyes tearing) . . . I don't really know if it's fear.		
Nurse: Ah huh. What *does* it feel like?		
(Silence.)		
Jennie: I guess . . . (silence, tearing, looking down into lap as though to attempt to compose herself).		
Nurse: You look so sad to me. Are you thinking about Scott and what's happening between you, when you speak of rejection?		
Jennie (crying): I don't think I can talk about that (looking very sad, tears coming down her cheeks but with no sobbing —very controlled crying).		

INTERACTION (VERBAL AND NONVERBAL)	NURSE-CENTERED ANALYSIS	CLIENT-CENTERED ANALYSIS
Nurse: It's really hard for you to talk about it, I see. (Pause.) Nurse: Are you able to cry about it sometimes? Jennie (softly): Yeah, at home I can. Nurse: How is it for you? Jennie (softly): I don't know . . . I guess it . . . it helps sometimes. (Pause.) A lot of times when he was there though, I couldn't. Nurse: When he was there you couldn't cry? Jennie (continues quietly): Yeah, because he never . . . always . . . I don't know . . . he just never liked to see me cry. He'd leave the room or something, or . . . or I'd go in the bedroom . . . . He'd just never like to see me cry. Or if he'd see me . . . if I was crying . . . during the nervous breakdown he'd . . . he'd just, um, he'd just shake his head and walk away. Nurse: You had to keep your crying—and feelings—from him. He acted as though your way of trying to communicate feelings was a sign of . . . weakness? Jennie: Yes! And he'd act like		

INTERACTION (VERBAL AND NONVERBAL)	NURSE-CENTERED ANALYSIS	CLIENT-CENTERED ANALYSIS
it was just a sign of a breakdown. Nurse: That must have been so painful, to have to keep so many feelings inside. . . . What things were you feeling that were making you sad? Jennie: What I was going through . . . what I was going through during the nervous breakdown and . . . and also the fact that . . . (long pause) that he wasn't there to reassure me or anything (voice fragile). Nurse: That you were alone in this. Jennie: Yes. And instead of reassuring me he just went the other way . . . started to shake his head at me. Put me down for it. He . . . I don't think he did that right at the beginning but he . . . (quietly) he finally did it. Nurse: So . . . you were holding your feelings in, because they were making it hard on him? Jenning (cuts in): Maybe. Because, I guess, it's because, not because it was . . . hard on him . . . it's because whenever I did it . . . he'd look down on me, you know. Nurse: What do you think he was thinking? Looking down on you. Jennie: That I was . . .		

INTERACTION (VERBAL AND NONVERBAL)	NURSE-CENTERED ANALYSIS	CLIENT-CENTERED ANALYSIS
incapable and . . . weak and not happy and . . . Nurse: Because you were crying? Jennie: Well, not just the crying, it was like he'd see me . . . into the nervous . . . thing of the nervous breakdown, you know, where I seem to be compelled to wash my hands, something like that . . . because, I had fears and I wasn't thinking very . . . I don't know . . . it was all . . . it was all the fears. Nurse: Um hum. Jennie: But I never realized it when I was having a nervous breakdown, but, everything that, um, everything . . . the four main things that I had with the nervous breakdown were. . . . Um . . . I think (looking at tape recorder), I think it's bothering me to have that on. Nurse: Oh. Well, maybe it's best that we talk about it, if you feel that it's difficult. Are there things you wanted to say that you're hesitating? Jennie: Well. What were we talking about? Nurse: You were about to tell me that there were four things . . . about the nervous breakdown.		

INTERACTION (VERBAL AND NONVERBAL)	NURSE-CENTERED ANALYSIS	CLIENT-CENTERED ANALYSIS
Jennie: Oh yeah, after I found out—like a couple of years later—that I had low blood sugar, um, after reading some of the things the doctor gave me and then . . . um, some of the . . . a book I had on it . . . those four things were . . . well, they could be symptoms of other things but they're also symptoms of low blood sugar. . . . And the doctor never tested me for low blood sugar.		
Nurse: When you had the nervous breakdown?		
Jennie: Yeah, they never did.		
Nurse: Are you wondering now, if, when you had the breakdown, if it could have been caused by the low blood sugar—if, because there wasn't a test done at that time, . . .		
Jennie: Wait, I'm lost at the beginning.		
Nurse: Are you thinking now that the breakdown might have been caused by low blood sugar?		
Jennie: I'm thinking it could have been.		
Nurse: That's something you're questioning. . . . Um, I don't . . . I can't give you an answer for that, but I think what you're going . . .		
Jennie (cuts in): You know		

INTERACTION (VERBAL AND NONVERBAL)	NURSE-CENTERED ANALYSIS	CLIENT-CENTERED ANALYSIS
(laugh), that tape recorder bothers me. Nurse: Okay. Let's turn it off. (Turns off tape.) (In the remainder of the session, Jennie related her fears of being seen as "crazy" and of feeling "crazy." She discussed her mother's long history of "crazy" behavior. Jennie fears a sick label for herself.)		

Analyzing a Group Session

DIRECTIONS

Analyze the following verbatim recording of a session of an ongoing outpatient psychotherapy group led by cotherapists. In making your analysis, refer to activity 41, "Guide to Interaction Process Analysis."

The group members are:

Janeen, thirty-three-year-old housewife, with three children, ages four, two and a half, and sixteen months. She has held several low-paying, low-status jobs during her married years. She expresses herself by complete submissiveness, and is fearful of losing control of the intense rage she feels. Janeen has a low self-concept and low self-esteem and cries frequently. She wants to find herself but fears that in doing so she may have to make some decisions regarding her marital situation. Although Janeen describes her marriage as intolerable, she states she loves her husband and wants to preserve the marriage. She has made one suicide attempt.

Linda, thirty-five-year-old housewife, with three children, ages nine, six, and four. Linda has never worked outside the home. She has often threatened her alcoholic husband with separation but is unable to carry through. She reacts to multiple humiliations with either passivity or rage. Linda is terrified to live alone, sure that she cannot support herself and the children. She is unaware of her legal rights regarding alimony and property division. She has a poor self-concept and low self-esteem and wants to develop confidence in herself.

Mary Ann, fifty-two-year-old widow, with four married children and one sixteen-year-old daughter. This daughter was turned away from the home because she was unmanageable. Mary Ann is depressed, feels worthless, and has little hope that things will ever change. At thirty-five years of age she suffered a heart attack and was told by her physician that she was disabled. Mary Ann is submissive in all problem situations, describing herself as a doormat. She often feels suicidal but has not made an attempt.

Lisa, twenty-two-year-old housewife, who holds a full-time job as a graphic artist. Lisa lived with her husband for four years before they married. She professes to adhere to modern views on life, but finds herself powerless within the confines of her marriage. Lisa admits to severe marital difficulties but is unable to consider living alone. She is depressed and thinks of suicide but has not made any attempts. Lisa feels isolated and alienated, believing that others will not understand her. Her feeling of self-worth is low.

Nancy, the fifth member of the group, who did not attend the session or call to say that she wouldn't be able to come.

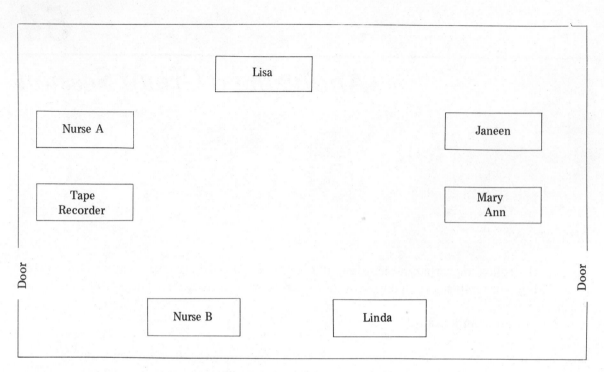

Figure 2. Seating chart, group therapy session 2

Interaction Process Analysis

INTERACTION (VERBAL AND NONVERBAL)	NURSE-CENTERED ANALYSIS	CLIENT-CENTERED ANALYSIS
Mary Ann: I've been doing a lot of thinking about this group this past week. Could you tell me what this group is supposed to do for you anyway? Nurse B: I wonder if anyone might want to help Mary Ann out with that? Janeen: I think it's been too easy for us to dwell only on ourselves. After a while, I begin to think I'm the only one that has any problems. Being in this		

INTERACTION (VERBAL AND NONVERBAL)	NURSE-CENTERED ANALYSIS	CLIENT-CENTERED ANALYSIS
group is showing me that I'm not the only one with a problem. (Others nod in agreement.) Linda: Maybe it's easier to say things here that maybe you wouldn't say anywhere else. Lisa: It's been important for me to see that other people can have problems. I agree that it's pretty easy to sit and feel sorry for yourself . . . as if nobody can be as miserable as you. Nurse B: A group like this can give people an opportunity to look at each other and look at themselves in an open and honest way. It could give you a better understanding of your relationships with other people. Nurse A: Yes. It can also be a safe place to say things and try different ways of handling problems. Mary Ann: I have something I'd like to try out on the group. My sister-in-law sent me an invitation to a luncheon. She's the sort of person who knows everybody, and everything has to be the best. I am not going to go. (There is a little flurry of activity, and several people speak in unison.) Lisa: I don't think you should		

INTERACTION (VERBAL AND NONVERBAL)	NURSE-CENTERED ANALYSIS	CLIENT-CENTERED ANALYSIS
stay away just because they have more than you do. Just because they have more money than you doesn't mean they are better than you. I think you should go. You might have a good time. Janeen: Having money doesn't mean much. I know a man who has a lot of money and is as nice as anyone could want. But then, there is another man who has a lot of money. He is an executive and has everything anyone could want. He is as nasty as can be. So, I don't think it makes any difference how much money anyone has. You're just as good as they are. I think you should go, too. Linda: Sure you should go. You can't just sit home and feel sorry for yourself. Just go. After you're there for a while, I bet you'll forget about it and have a good time. Mary Ann: But the money doesn't bother me. I don't think they are better than me. It's something else and I don't know what it is. Guilt I guess. I always feel guilty. Maybe they'll reject me. (Again the members try to give her support and encouragement. The group is talking spontaneously and the atmosphere is one of support and good feelings for each other.)		

INTERACTION (VERBAL AND NONVERBAL)	NURSE-CENTERED ANALYSIS	CLIENT-CENTERED ANALYSIS
Janeen (to Mary Ann): You know, I've been thinking about you this week. You are in a position to be able to do anything you want to. With no husband or kids to take care of, you . . . you could even go back to school, or get a job.		
Mary Ann: I've worked before. I worked for years at Community Hospital, but I don't know if I could do it physically.		
Lisa: They have some really interesting courses at the university that you could look into.		
Mary Ann: I don't know. Maybe I can't do it. What if I can't make it?		
Linda: You can always start easy. Look into the credit-free programs at the university. They cost very little money, and, if you are worried about failing or not doing well, they won't be marking you.		
Mary Ann: I don't know. It just seems so hard to do. Tell me, how do you go about it? How do you change your life?		
Linda: You just do it! You do it one step at a time.		
Janeen: No one else can do it for you. We can only give you suggestions, but you have to do it.		

INTERACTION (VERBAL AND NONVERBAL)	NURSE-CENTERED ANALYSIS	CLIENT-CENTERED ANALYSIS
(Lisa nods in agreement.) (The group gradually became more silent as Mary Ann continued to block their suggestions. She then dominated the session with stories of her failure as a mother—her youngest son and daughter have been in a lot of trouble. She went on to discuss the many severe beatings her youngest daughter had at the hands of other family members.) Mary Ann: I didn't hit her. I never stopped them either. I just stood by and let them beat her. Of course at the time I was very angry too. Was I wrong? (Silence.) Nurse B: I wonder if the group might try to answer Mary Ann. Linda: Well, I think you were wrong. Maybe you were not involved, but you let it go on. (Mary Ann continued to be verbally active, while the other members became more and more silent. Nurse A: I notice how different this meeting is from the last meeting. I'm wondering what you think the difference might be. . . . These silences seem very uncomfortable. (Silence.)		

INTERACTION (VERBAL AND NONVERBAL)	NURSE-CENTERED ANALYSIS	CLIENT-CENTERED ANALYSIS
Nurse B: Mary Ann seems to be blocking all your suggestions for help. That must be frustrating for the person who is trying to help. (Silence.) (Mary Ann began talking again about being afraid to go out socially. She believes people are talking about her because of all the "bad things" her children have done—their trouble with the law.) Linda (emphatically): Well, I think that's very unreasonable. My husband is a heavy drinker and has done many things to embarrass me, but I no longer assume any responsibility for his actions. (An extremely long silence— four or five minutes.) Janeen: I don't want to take up too much time talking about myself, but there is one thing I would like to say. I saw my father a few weeks ago for the first time in about thirteen years. It was really nice. Better than it's ever been. He's been in Florida. He brought me frozen shrimp and lobster, and they were just great. He said, "The one thing I really feel bad about is the fact that your mother never loved you." So that's all I am going to say. (Another silence. Mary Ann		

INTERACTION (VERBAL AND NONVERBAL)	NURSE-CENTERED ANALYSIS	CLIENT-CENTERED ANALYSIS
occasionally began talking but eventually became silent. This silence also lasted for four or five minutes. Janeen was tearful and appeared angry and/or sad.)		
Nurse A: There is definitely something going on here, even though it's silent. As I look around, I can see some sad faces, and I see some angry faces.		
Mary Ann: Maybe we need some humor around here. Has anyone heard about the traveling salesman?		
Linda: No, Mary Ann. What is it?		
Mary Ann: I guess I forgot it.		
Janeen: Knock, knock!		
Mary Ann: Who's there?		
Janeen: Sarah.		
Mary Ann: Sarah, who?		
Janeen: Sarah Doctor in the house?		
(Polite laughs around the room. Again the group reverted to silence. The tension seemed to mount, and finally Janeen stood up.)		
Janeen (briskly): Children are sweet and innocent things. I am going home. (She got her hat and coat and left.)		

INTERACTION (VERBAL AND NONVERBAL)	NURSE-CENTERED ANALYSIS	CLIENT-CENTERED ANALYSIS
Nurse B: I'm feeling surprised that Janeen would leave without explaining to us why she felt she needed to go. I wonder how everyone is feeling about this?		
Lisa: I had a feeling that she didn't want to be here in the first place.		
Mary Ann: I just have this feeling that somehow I chased her away. I feel responsible.		
Nurse A: When a member leaves or is missing, it affects the whole group.		
Linda: I think that the girl who is not here (referring to Nancy) is different though. She never said anything to us. We didn't know anything about her.		
Mary Ann: I think Janeen left because she told us too much about herself last week. I think she felt too uncomfortable with us.		
Nurse B: Mary Ann, you have told us a great deal about yourself tonight.		
Mary Ann: Well, I'll be here next week. I gave you my commitment for the next twelve weeks, and I'll be here.		
Lisa: You know, I've been thinking whether this group is right for me or not. I heard there is a group of younger		

INTERACTION (VERBAL AND NONVERBAL)	NURSE-CENTERED ANALYSIS	CLIENT-CENTERED ANALYSIS
people here, but then . . . I don't know whether that would be right either. It doesn't seem as if my problems have anything in common with any of you women. My lifestyle is very different. Mary Ann: Maybe I'm older than you, but what makes you think you won't be in the same position as I am when you are my age? We're all the same. Lisa: Well, for one thing, I won't have six kids. Mary Ann: Do you think I'm going to treat you like a mother would? Lisa: You already have. Mary Ann: What do you mean? How? Lisa: For one thing, you were very upset when you talked about your daughter smoking pot. I smoke pot, and I don't think I'm terrible. (Both Mary Ann and Linda laugh loudly.) Linda: I hate to disillusion you but I've smoked pot lots of times before. Lisa (clearly shocked): But I mean on a regular basis. Linda: The only reason I don't smoke more often is that I just		

INTERACTION (VERBAL AND NONVERBAL)	NURSE-CENTERED ANALYSIS	CLIENT-CENTERED ANALYSIS
don't like it. It's not that big of a deal, you know. (The group paused, seeming to consider what had just occurred.) Nurse A: We only have about five minutes left. Maybe we could spend the time talking about what happened tonight and how you feel about it. Lisa: I know things are a little better for me, but I don't know what I can do about my mother-in-law. I think she is my biggest problem now. (Lisa then goes into specific detail on how she has been mistreated by her mother-in-law and made to be a pawn in the battle between mother and son.) Nurse B: So, it seems then, that, although the problems one has may be different from someone else's, the pain they cause isn't. Nurse A: Maybe the way that people respond to their problems might be important in learning how to make things easier. The problems may be different but feelings are shared by everyone. (Again a silence, but the tension that was present earlier was absent.)		

INTERACTION (VERBAL AND NONVERBAL)	NURSE-CENTERED ANALYSIS	CLIENT-CENTERED ANALYSIS
Nurse B: I want to remind you all that membership in the group is open, and there may be new members next week. (At this point, people began to leave the room.)		

Analyzing Marital Couple Interaction

DIRECTIONS

Analyze the following verbatim recording of a second session with a couple in marital therapy. In making your analysis, refer to activity 41, "Guide to Interaction Process Analysis."

Tom and Karen have been married for twelve years. Karen had telephoned the mental health agency because of "serious marital problems" that needed to be talked about. They have an eleven-year-old son, Mark, but did not wish to include him in sessions at this time due to the "urgent" and "adult" nature of the problems.

Tom had a medical history of a spontaneous pneumothorax four years ago and has suffered terrible coughing spasms since then. The episode altered his view on life toward "getting all the enjoyment I can—I could probably drop dead any time!"

During the week following the first therapy session, Karen called saying that they had again talked and that Tom had "let it all out." He told her he had an extramarital relationship of two years' standing. On the phone with Karen the nurse suggested the three of them talk about this at the next session.

INTERACTION (VERBAL AND NONVERBAL)	NURSE-CENTERED ANALYSIS	CLIENT-CENTERED ANALYSIS
Nurse: Let's see . . . I talked with you, Karen, on Thursday.		
Karen: Yes, Thursday night.		
(Silence.)		
Nurse: Karen let me know, Tom, that you and she had had a further conversation the night after our first meeting.		

INTERACTION (VERBAL AND NONVERBAL)	NURSE-CENTERED ANALYSIS	CLIENT-CENTERED ANALYSIS
Tom: Um hum.		
Nurse: . . . and that you had shared with her the fact that you have been involved with another woman. Karen told me of this briefly, over the phone. I asked her if she could talk about it here, instead, as I want our work together to take place when we're all here, so that we all have the same base to work from.		
Tom: Yes, she told me she had talked with you. (Monotone, low voice. Contrasts with his "cocky" manner the week before.)		
(Silence.)		
Nurse: Maybe there are things either of you would like to share here		
Karen: Why don't you start? (Looks to Tom.)		
Tom: You start—go ahead.		
(Pause.)		
Tom: I don't know what to say. You go ahead.		
Nurse: Kind of hard to talk about things?		
Karen: Well, I explained to her (looking at Tom) about your friend . . .		
Tom: Um hum.		

INTERACTION (VERBAL AND NONVERBAL)	NURSE-CENTERED ANALYSIS	CLIENT-CENTERED ANALYSIS
Karen: . . . and I asked her if she felt we should continue with this. And . . . ah . . . she said . . . we should . . . and that . . . whatever happens we'd have to prepare Mark for this. Tom: Um hum. Karen: 'Cause he's part of this family. Tom: Right. Karen: So . . . that's that. (Silence.) Nurse: I guess I'm thinking—not only to prepare Mark, but for yourselves too—it may be useful to talk more on what you have begun. I'm thinking that sometimes moves are made impulsively. It may be that you aren't looking to a separation, for instance . . . or that you may want time to think about it. How is it for you? Tom: Right! . . . Ah, I would like time to think this over. To see if it's what I really want to do. . . . Ah . . . This friend of mine, I . . . I don't expect to marry . . . at least I don't think so, not right away. . . . It's just that . . . well . . . we get along together real well. Of course we don't live together. I suppose if we did maybe we'd find fault in one another . . . like when, you know, when you're married to someone!		

INTERACTION (VERBAL AND NONVERBAL)	NURSE-CENTERED ANALYSIS	CLIENT-CENTERED ANALYSIS
Nurse: Things about being married make it somewhat different?		
Tom: Yeah . . . yeah. Just like, well, after we got married we found out things about one another that . . . while they looked real rosy before we got married . . . then it's not quite so good afterwards.		
Nurse: How about that, Karen, how's it been for you?		
Karen: Well, you can't just have all sweetness and light when you're married. Somebody's got to take care of things. . . . Things do change . . .		
Tom (interrupts): But . . . ah . . . rather than just move out tomorrow . . . I would like some time to think about it and . . . if I do move out . . . ah . . . we would have to come to an amicable agreement or understanding. So that neither one of us gets taken to the dry cleaners . . . or . . . gets hurt. But . . . it's something that should take time and consideration to think about.		
Nurse: Are you asking Karen for some time to think things through?		
Tom: Yeah.		
Nurse (gestures toward Karen): Can you ask her directly?		

INTERACTION (VERBAL AND NONVERBAL)	NURSE-CENTERED ANALYSIS	CLIENT-CENTERED ANALYSIS
Tom: Oh . . . yeah. . . . I . . . I wish we . . . could think about this . . . before making any decisions. . . . (Pause.) Maybe it's just the idea that I would like my freedom, so that I can do as I please without hurting her.		
Nurse: Who?		
Tom: Oh . . . hurting you (to Karen) or Mark or . . . having a guilt complex about it. I just . . . if I want to . . . stay out late or go someplace . . . I don't want to have to be responsible to her . . . (low voice) to anyone but myself.		
Karen: (Loud coughing.)		
Nurse (looking to Karen): You'd like to respond to Tom?		
Karen (speaking rapidly): You mean when he first told me about this? (Seems to be attempting to control anger.)		
Nurse: Or now?		
Karen: Well . . . I feel if that's what he wants he should have it! If he wants his freedom—and feels that there isn't enough happiness here—I feel that's due him. Just as it's due me. I mean it wouldn't be fair for me to take it away from him, and it wouldn't be fair for him to take it away from me.		

INTERACTION (VERBAL AND NONVERBAL)	NURSE-CENTERED ANALYSIS	CLIENT-CENTERED ANALYSIS
Nurse: I'm puzzled. Go on with that a bit in terms of how it is for you. Karen: Well . . . I've had my suspicions . . . and I felt that there would come a time when he would just . . . tell me. And I felt . . . well, why . . . push the issue. . . . When the time is right, he'll just . . . cough it up! (Blows smoke in his direction.) (The rest of the time was spent planning future sessions. The three agreed to focus on getting in touch with the anger and hurt each partner had experienced.)		

Analyzing Family Interaction

DIRECTIONS

Analyze the following verbatim recording of this family therapy session. In making your analysis, refer to activity 41, "Guide to Interaction Process Analysis."

The James family was referred for counseling by an agency for retarded children with whom the family has contact. Mrs. James had expressed concern about the future of the marriage and the welfare of her children because of the conflict between her and her husband around matters of discipline. She believed the problem to be a result of his verbal abuse of her and his physical abuse of the children. Mr. James was an angry, rigid, and extremely suspicious man who believed that their problems arose from his wife's attitude toward his authority and her refusal to have a sexual relationship with him. Shortly after the second therapy session with the marital couple, Mr. James moved out of the house. Within a few more weeks, he had severed direct communication with all members of the family.

The family members are:

Dave James, the father, thirty-five years old. Three years ago he injured his back and was no longer able to continue his work as a landscape gardener. His behavior toward the children, especially the two boys, has become more violent since this time. He now works as a mail sorter.

Nancy James, thirty-four, the mother and housewife. She is a high school graduate who has not worked outside of the home since her marriage.

Jeff, the twelve-year-old son. He is a sixth-grade student who was held back in school one year for underachievement. Almost immediately after his father's departure from the home, Jeff's school work began to improve. He is not developmentally disabled.

Jimmy, the eight-year-old son. He is a second-grader, also held back one year for underachievement.

Karen, the seven-year-old daughter. She is in first grade and, like her brothers, was held back one year for underachievement.

Cora, the four-year-old daughter. She is severely developmentally disabled and requires total care. She lives at home.

This is the first session with the family and without the father. The nurse has arranged to come to the James house.

Interaction Process Analysis

INTERACTION (VERBAL AND NONVERBAL)	NURSE-CENTERED ANALYSIS	CLIENT-CENTERED ANALYSIS
(When the nurse arrived, Nancy looked quite tired and bedraggled but the house was neat and clean. Jeff was sitting at the dining room table doing homework. When the nurse invited him to join the group, he said he was much too busy. The nurse sat down on the living room couch, and the children milled about the room. Nancy also sat on the couch. The nurse showed them the tape recorder.) Nurse: Do you know what this is? Jimmy: See! I told you, Mom! Nancy: Tell the lady what you told me, Jimmy. Jimmy: I knew she'd have a tape recorder. Nancy: Well, go on! Jimmy (somewhat reluctantly): I told Mom you'd tape us and then let Dad hear it. (The nurse then explained the terms of confidentiality very clearly and told why she liked to use a tape recorder during a family meeting. She explained that after reviewing the tape she would erase it. The family		

INTERACTION (VERBAL AND NONVERBAL)	NURSE-CENTERED ANALYSIS	CLIENT-CENTERED ANALYSIS
seemed satisfied with this.) Nurse: I've already told you who I am and what I do. What I'd like to do now is hear from all of you about what you think is happening in your family? Karen: I think it's all wrong. Nurse: You think it's all wrong? Jimmy (very carefully enunciating): He's mixed up in the head. Right, Jeff? Karen: Yeah, he's blaming it all on Mommy, and it ain't true. He's doing . . . Jimmy (interrupts): Yeah, he's making up stuff. Nurse: Wait—wait. Let's try and set up a rule for our meetings. If someone is talking, let's wait until they're finished. Everyone will get a chance to talk. Jimmy: You mean raise our hand? Nurse: No. But if Karen is talking, wait until she is finished before you talk. Now, Karen, you were saying Dad is blaming everything on Mom, and it's all wrong. Karen: Yeah. And, he's hitting us too hard. He's hitting us in the head and it might		

INTERACTION (VERBAL AND NONVERBAL)	NURSE-CENTERED ANALYSIS	CLIENT-CENTERED ANALYSIS
damage our head. That ain't right to hit us in the face or the head.		
Jimmy: For one thing, he gave me a black eye already, and—this is kinda funny—my father pushed Jeff into the window (laughs).		
Nurse: What do you mean?		
Jimmy and Karen (talking at once): The big window in Jeff's room got broken.		
(Jimmy got up to demonstrate how his father pushed Jeff into the window, breaking it.)		
Nurse: You really think that's funny?		
Jimmy: No, not when it happened.		
Karen (speaking at the same time): No.		
Nurse: I don't see it as funny either.		
Jimmy: He says he believes in violence.		
Nurse: Is that the word he used?		
Jimmy: Yeah. He believes in violence. He says if you go out and play, and if anyone picks on you, break his jaw, and then go home, do your work, watch TV, and maybe play outside,		

INTERACTION (VERBAL AND NONVERBAL)	NURSE-CENTERED ANALYSIS	CLIENT-CENTERED ANALYSIS
and then go to bed. That's the way the day is supposed to go. . . . And working. . . . One little thing that Jeff and I do wrong, like take out the garbage, he smacks us. We go flying. Nurse: Gee, I wonder how you can take out the garbage wrong. Jimmy: He says there is only one way to do things—his way. Nurse: Do you believe there is only one way to do things? Jimmy and Karen: No. Karen: Plus, one night, um, um, you know, I didn't hear my mother cause I couldn't hear right and he kept smacking me until I did hear right. Like I was just sitting there eating my egg and my Mom was talking to me, but I didn't hear her. He screamed at me and kept hitting. Jimmy: Yeah. There's not one day that he doesn't smack me. I do something wrong, and he smacks me. Nurse: What kinds of things do you do wrong? Jimmy: He thinks when I come down the street, I stare at him and stuff. He thinks I'm a jerk. He's the jerk! I gotta tell you something: me and Karen were laying down watching TV like this (demonstrates how they		

INTERACTION (VERBAL AND NONVERBAL)	NURSE-CENTERED ANALYSIS	CLIENT-CENTERED ANALYSIS
were lying on the floor), just watching TV happily, and he comes along, kicks me and Karen in the back for no reason. "Get out of the way" (gruffly imitates father). Karen: Yeah, and we didn't even see him. Jimmy: Bam! "Get out of the way!" Karen: Then he kicked me in the spine and that really hurt. Nurse: Wow, how does that make you feel? Karen: I feel terrible. Jimmy: When I get bigger, oh, man! He's going to have a busted jaw. I'm going to get him back. Jeff (cries out): I'll smash him! Nurse: What was that, Jeff? Jeff: I didn't say anything. (He appeared to be quite busy with his work.) (Nancy took Cora upstairs and put her to bed, while the other children continued to talk. The nurse generally kept the talk on a superficial level, because she wanted Nancy present when the children were ventilating their feelings and experiences with their father. When Nancy returned, the nurse encouraged		

INTERACTION (VERBAL AND NONVERBAL)	NURSE-CENTERED ANALYSIS	CLIENT-CENTERED ANALYSIS
them to continue discussing their feelings about their father.) Karen: Well, the first time he left, I cried and cried. I couldn't stop. It just went on and on. But, you know, now it's better. It's so much better since he's gone. Jimmy: Yeah. Me and Jeff used to listen to him holler at Mom about her "games." He used to say that Mom was playing bedtime games. Nurse: Boy, sounds like you kids know a lot about what was going on between Mom and Dad. Jimmy: Sure we do. Karen (simultaneously): We're in the family. Nurse: Nancy, did you know that Karen and Jimmy were aware of the problems between you and Dave? Nancy (stammering): Well, I, I knew they knew something, but I guess not really so much. Jimmy: In the middle of the day, he screamed at Mom, and the screen door was open. And he used to smack Jeff right out in the open. He smacks me out in the open, and everybody stares. Karen: And you know what?		

INTERACTION (VERBAL AND NONVERBAL)	NURSE-CENTERED ANALYSIS	CLIENT-CENTERED ANALYSIS
Daddy pushed Mommy into the bushes one time. Nurse: Sounds like some pretty scary things have been happening here. Karen: Yeah. You should love your children. You should treat them right. When you have a life like this, you can't teach your children nothing. When you have problems, you can't do nothing. Jimmy: I know. Nurse: An example would help me get a clearer picture of what you mean. Karen: I mean when they're screaming at each other, I can't do nothing. I can't even play a game. It gets so scary. Jimmy: The other night we watched that movie about that man that beat his wife, and he threw the boy across the room. And then the lady lied about it. Boy, she shouldn't have lied about it. *I would not stick up for him!* (Said with emphasis.) (Jeff at this began to join the conversation, from the dining room, adding comments particularly of hate and vengeance toward the father.) Jeff: Dad is just like his own father, [the children's grandfather]. Mean and nasty.		

INTERACTION (VERBAL AND NONVERBAL)	NURSE-CENTERED ANALYSIS	CLIENT-CENTERED ANALYSIS
I know because my grandmother told me so. (The children began to talk among themselves, trying to think of possible explanations for their father's behavior. Jimmy felt that his father must have had high blood pressure to act the way he did. Jeff became very interested at this point.) Jeff (from dining room): It wouldn't make any difference what Dad did. He could go to the best psychiatrist in the world, but he will *never* change. Jimmy: He used to yell at her all the time because she wouldn't go dancing. Karen: Yeah. She ain't interested in that. That's crazy. Nurse: She isn't interested in what? Karen: Sex. Nurse: I wonder. Is that true, Mom? Karen (quite surprised): Are you? Nancy (laughs and then replies): Well, sure I am. Sex is an important part of a good relationship between a man and a woman. Jimmy: And Dad thinks me and Jeff are homosexuals. He said he caught me and Jeff fagging		

INTERACTION (VERBAL AND NONVERBAL)	NURSE-CENTERED ANALYSIS	CLIENT-CENTERED ANALYSIS
off. He's crazy—that ain't true. Nurse: You know what? I see you smiling, but I have a feeling you're not really smiling underneath. Jimmy: Not really, no! Man, he has no reason to say that. That's not true. He has no right to say that. (The discussion continued with more and more disclosures of beatings, hurts, and humiliations. Jeff joined in more and more. After about forty-five minutes, he left his work in the dining room to join the family in the living room.)		